Wait Until You're Fifty

A Woman's Journey Into Midlife

To Chris –

Wishing you a great journey!

Mindy

Wait Until You're Fifty

A Woman's Journey Into Midlife

Mindy Littman Holland

SANTA FE

Sunstone books may be purchased for educational, business, or sales promotional use.
For information please write: Special Markets Department, Sunstone Press,
P.O. Box 2321, Santa Fe, New Mexico 87504-2321.

Book and Cover design ✑ Vicki Ahl
Body typeface ✑ Book Antiqua
Printed on acid free paper

Library of Congress Cataloging-in-Publication Data

Holland, Mindy Littman, 1953-
  Wait until you're fifty : a woman's journey into midlife / by Mindy Littman Holland.
    p. cm.
  ISBN 978-0-86534-843-1 (sosftcover : alk. paper)
  1. Middle-aged women. 2. Middle-aged women--Psychology. 3. Women--Psychology.
I. Title.
  HQ1059.4.H65 2011
  305.244'2--dc23

                        2011036081

WWW.SUNSTONEPRESS.COM
SUNSTONE PRESS / POST OFFICE BOX 2321 / SANTA FE, NM 87504-2321 /USA
(505) 988-4418 / ORDERS ONLY (800) 243-5644 / FAX (505) 988-1025

*D*edicated to my parents,
Ralph and Gladys Littman,
who started me on this journey.

Contents

Introduction

❧❧

I've given a lot of thought to the title of this book, but no sound bite could capture the horror (and sometimes, guarded optimism) of crossing over into this no-man's land of change and disorientation.

When I was forty-two, an older friend waggled an arthritic index finger in my smooth young face and said, "Wait until you're fifty."

"Mark my words," she said with a demonic glaze in her presbyopic eyes, "nothing in your life will ever feel good again."

"But Babs," I protested, "you're only forty-eight."

"I feel like I'm fifty," she said.

I felt like running out for an industrial-strength container of *malocchio* repellant. Maybe Babs had a lousy attitude. Maybe she was born fifty. I felt like I was twenty-two at forty-two. What difference could eight years make?

"What does fifty feel like?" I asked.

"It feels like midriff bulge. It feels like you have a pair of fuzzy earmuffs wrapped around your brain. It feels like you don't want to get out of bed in the morning. It feels like you can't look at your neck without thinking candied yams and cranberry sauce."

I couldn't relate. Nobody can unless they're experiencing it firsthand and I had eight years to go—or six, by Babs' calendar.

"How about your sex drive?" I asked, trying to get back onto familiar turf.

"Please," she said, "I'm Italian; but my German husband would rather dress up in a pink tutu and dance in clogs than have sex with me, so my drive has nowhere to go."

"Are you going through menopause?" I asked, whispering "menopause" as if it were a dirty word. My mother always told me that women routinely had nervous breakdowns during menopause. For that reason, I lived in fear of it since puberty, dreading the advent of my first hot flash, terrified that I would be one of those poor unfortunates that ended up playing soccer with their own breasts and sending money to televangelists.

"Hell, no," Babs said. "I had a hysterectomy at thirty-five and have been on estrogen ever since. Fifty just sucks, that's all there is to it. Your skin begins to sag, waiters call you 'ma'am' and don't get me started on my saddlebags. You'll see."

Babs is not typical, I reasoned to keep from panicking. Surely I knew other women Babs' age who were doing just fine.

My closest friend was Babs' age. Marion was beautiful, refined and successful and was married to a man ten years her junior. Of course, she did die of ovarian cancer a month after she turned forty-nine. Poor example. Maybe I should mention Carly. She was a well-traveled public speaker, sexy, adventurous. She learned that she had

MS as she was circling the bowl of fifty. Now, she worries about wheelchairs and incontinence — another poor example. Hmmm. A good example evades me, at least among my female friends.

Maybe it's not just women, I thought. Several years ago, an old boyfriend warned me of the sand trap that is fifty. He sounded just like a male version of Babs.

"I looked great until I turned fifty," he boasted. "Then, it all fell apart. Now, I look like Grandpa Walton. You'll see."

Maybe he exaggerated his decrepitude. The last time I saw this guy he was sixty and an oarsman on an Olympic crew team. He was engaged to marry a beautiful thirty-eight-year-old Brazilian who wanted to have his baby. Go figure. Can you imagine a reverse scenario for a sixty-year-old woman, outside of Sophia Loren? Sure — maybe if she's loaded and on the verge of death.

Don't get me wrong. I don't want to downplay the angst that some men experience at midlife. Men are somewhat more susceptible to coronaries and colon cancer than women. Some may have a moment of remorse about their career choice. Generally speaking, though, men get off a lot easier than women. They may buy a red Corvette or trade in their wife or find new employment. Some may put a little Grecian Formula in their hair, if they still have any, or pop Viagra, if they don't have a heart condition. But, then, they get on with it, usually without the aid of antipsychotic drugs.

That's not to say that middle-aged women don't get coronaries and colon cancer and career willies. They do. In addition, they get hot flashes, night sweats, insomnia, mood swings, wrinkles, brain fog, migraines, vaginal dryness, cellulite, porous bones, memory loss and yeast infections — at about the same time their kids leave home and their husbands go hunting for strange. Thank God there's no chocolate shortage.

Thirty years ago, I experienced a scene that stuck with me. I was visiting my dying grandmother at the hospital. I went into the visitors' lounge to collect myself. There was a woman of about fifty sitting there in a wheelchair amid her family. From what I was able to overhear, she had somehow managed to get run over by her own car. Here's what made the impression. At the top of her lungs, she kept screaming over and over, "I'm old. I'm old. I'm old." It was horrible...worse than listening to Babs on a good day.

I decided that I was not going to fall apart at fifty. Why should I? At forty-two, I was at the top of my game. I had an exciting career and a comfortable six-figure income. I was able to read menus from less than six feet away. My hair was an uninterrupted shade of mahogany. My husband made thrillingly inappropriate sexual remarks to me in front of our dumbfounded friends. Why should I feel like the Sword of Damocles was hanging over my head?

Why? Because I was a woman and fifty was closer than I thought...even closer than Babs thought.

I got my first hot flash when I was forty-four. I remember the exact moment it occurred. My husband and I were in bed at the San Francisco Hyatt. One minute I was in the crook of my husband's arm, enjoying the cool crispness of the sheet and the soapy clean scent of his skin. The next moment, I was soaked in sweat from the collarbone up, ejecting myself from my husband's embrace like he was the Prince of Darkness. It was the beginning of a whole new ballgame, and I didn't know the half of it.

There are scores of books on the market that claim the years past fifty can be a woman's most creative. An AARP magazine cover announced, "Sixty is the New Thirty." That's the good news and the bad news. It's great to know that all hope is not lost as you go into the back fifty.

On the other hand, if you drag yourself out of bed at five in the morning, soggy and exhausted after a sleepless night, you shouldn't have to feel like a failure because you're not up to discovering a cure for AIDS that day. What's the good of having all that sunshine blown up your skirt if you can no longer wear the four-inch spikes that go with it?

With the proper attitude and maintenance, fifty can be tolerable and maybe even fine, a time of reinvention and spiritual growth. However, it can also be a protracted journey through a seemingly endless wall of fire, no matter how brave and upbeat you pretend to be.

I've written this book to give voice to women who are *schvitzing* (sweating) their way through midlife—either literally and/or figuratively, as they change their perspectives on relationships, careers, healthcare, self-image and spirituality. I hope it gives you some comfort, lots of practical survival tips and a few laughs.

And, for those men who read this book, I hope it gives you some perspective on what makes middle-aged women tick—and sometimes explode.

In The Beginning

❊

*H*ave you ever had the feeling that everything is fine until it's not? Like when you're on the verge of the flu, for example. One minute, you're power jogging beside a river feeling like you could go for ten miles, easy; the next minute, you're coughing like a coal miner and down with a fever of a hundred and two that sidelines you for two weeks. It makes you wonder how long something insidious lies undetected in your system before it makes its disgusting "surprise" appearance and takes over your entire existence.

"But I was fine a minute ago," you protest feebly from beneath your down comforter between coughing spasms.

Not really.

Menopause doesn't happen abruptly either, even though it may seem that way. There's a long purgatorial period known as "perimenopause" that starts to bedevil some women as early as the thirties. It all has to do with a humorous little vaudeville team, known as estrogen and progesterone. This nefarious duo can create unbelievable havoc for a woman, especially when they begin to fluctuate themselves.

Think back to when you were going through puberty. In preparation for the joys of womanhood, your breasts began to hurt, you got migraines, you got bloated, you became moody, your skin broke out and you got strong sexual urges that you probably had to suppress for several years.

Then came the first period, the best and worst day of your young life. I personally woke up in agony and spent the next ten days hemorrhaging, but it was a great day for my mother. She chased me around the house to give me a ritual slap in the face before telling me I was now eligible to have a child. I was two weeks shy of my thirteenth birthday. Let the babies begin (actually, having sex was still *verboten*). When my father came running to find out what all the commotion was about, she whispered that I was 'unwell', the family euphemism for menstruating.

Yes, I felt unwell, thanks to those two newcomers in my life, estrogen and progesterone. But, I was also proud to be a woman, along with all the pain and discomfort that went with it. How exciting to be fertile and nubile, blossoming into adulthood with my whole life ahead of me. What could be more thrilling?

Menopause is like being on the wrong end of puberty. The hormones still rage because they're reluctant to leave, but leave they must. Unless you go through surgical menopause — a hysterectomy that includes the removal of the ovaries — the departure occurs over time. It's like moving out of a house you've lived in for decades. You don't transfer all of your belongings into your downsized digs all at once. You move one box at a time.

By the time some women get to the end of their child bearing years, they can't wait to see the end of their periods. That's largely because estrogen and progesterone can get very surly towards the end of a woman's reproductive life. They can make you bleed too much or too little or too unexpectedly. They can trick you into thinking you can no longer conceive. Then, you end up getting pregnant at forty-eight, which can be particularly appalling if your husband's had a vasectomy.

I am not enthusiastic about losing my periods. I look forward to their demise about as much as I look forward to finding my first gray pubic hair. I figure as long as I'm bleeding, I'm getting some protection against osteoporosis and heart disease, not to mention sexual undesirability.

I read somewhere that men of all ages are attracted to ovulating women, something having to do with the propagation of the species. When I miss a period, I still rush out for a pregnancy test, preferring to believe that I'm pregnant (even though my husband had a vasectomy thirty years ago) than accept that I'm menopausal. But, hey, now that I'm (holy shit) fifty, I'm going to have to face reality — in the not-too-distant future, I will be officially too old to reproduce.

Yet, the realization takes its time sinking in. Two days after my fiftieth birthday, I was racing down the highway trying to pass a truck. I was on my way to a drugstore to buy what I told myself would be my last pregnancy test. What the hell — my period was three months overdue and I was getting frequent nosebleeds. Nosebleeds probably didn't count as a symptom of pregnancy, but I didn't want to take any chances. I gave up on trying to pass the truck and got behind him to get off at my exit. On the back on the vehicle was a sign bearing the following words: "The Rabbit is Alive!" I saluted the driver and said, "Thank you, buddy, you just saved me fifteen bucks."

Speak of getting a message from the universe. And yet, two days later, I ended up taking a pregnancy test, anyway. It confirmed that I was…insane! If I'd passed a billboard on the way to the drugstore that screamed, "Get Your Head Examined," maybe I would've saved another fifteen bucks. I doubt it, though. I took another test the next day. It doesn't hurt to get a second opinion. It confirmed that I was… ugly, too! Thank you, Rodney Dangerfield.

The Permanently Empty Nest

※3※

$\mathscr{I}$ got a reflexology massage at my health club. The reflexologist kneaded a portion of my foot that caused me to ooh and ah with pleasure.

"What organ does that part of my foot correspond with?" I asked.

"It's your uterus," she replied, and then added, "Reproduction is what it's all about for women."

If I weren't enjoying having my uterus stroked so much, I probably would've leaped out of the chair and said, "Speak for yourself, sister." It was so politically incorrect. On the other hand, it was so realistically dead on.

Some women know for certain that they want children. When they're little girls playing house, they plan to have gobs of children when they grow up. They may also plan to be ballerinas or astronauts or brain surgeons, but reproduction takes precedence over everything else. Even if they grow up to be gay, sexual orientation does not interfere with the drive toward motherhood.

Some women have children because they're sixteen and they happen to be in the back seat of a Buick with an over-eager boy who either doesn't want to or doesn't know how to wear a rubber. Some have children because it's expected of them. Some have children late in life at great expense and sacrifice to their health because they feel like they're missing the boat if they don't. Some women are dead-set against having children. We think of them as selfish bitches — or career girls.

Then, there are women who seem to be ambivalent about children. They secretly want them but suppress their desire because they don't want to be a single parent or they're with a mate who doesn't want children or they have a uterus that feels great but doesn't work.

I have friends that always knew they wanted children. They found a willing, like-minded mate early in the game, got married, got their masters degree in anthropology, put their husbands through medical school and spawned. They loved the carpooling, the soccer games, the Girl Scout cookie drives and the clamor and chaos of childrearing. Their nests were empty before they even made it to midlife.

So, what do they do? They sell real estate, take tennis lessons, get tummy tucks, do volunteer work and wait for their children to have children so they can start all over again doing the only thing that's ever mattered to them. What about the husband? He's off having an affair with the selfish bitch that chose a career over getting stretch marks and dodging projectile baby vomit.

The women who got pregnant at sixteen either had abortions, gave the babies up for adoption, dropped out of high school and had several more babies, or got married and had "legitimate" children, whether they wanted them or not. The ones who chose to give their babies up and never have another are the ones with the biggest regrets. They are full of "what ifs" as they rattle around in their empty nests; no matter how well their lives have turned out and how great a relationship they've got with their partners.

Women who have children because they feel like they must are most often resentful of both their spouses and their children, especially female children. They dislike making the sacrifices having children requires because they didn't really want the burden from the start. Sons they can tolerate because, while they can be irritating like their fathers, they are non-threatening—unlike daughters, who are becoming ovulating hotties at the same time their mothers are falling into the dried-out midlife abyss.

Are such mothers proud of their sparkling superstar daughters? Absolutely, because they reflect what the mother once was or wanted to be. Are such mothers also shamefully jealous of their nubile daughters? You bet they are. Bring on the empty nest!

What about that selfish bitch that knows she doesn't want to have children? Perhaps she's not so selfish after all. Not everybody is cut out to be a mother and it's a shame that not more women know that.

Becoming Invisible

※∺※

*H*ave you noticed that the older you get, the less visible you become? I'm not talking melting sensation like the one experienced by the dowsed Wicked Witch of the West; I'm talking a disappearing act in which you appear visible only to yourself and similarly afflicted aging females. Perhaps it is awareness that men are no longer seeing you or, worse yet, that the only men that appear to be seeing you are thirty years your senior.

If you are accustomed to garnering a lot of attention from the opposite sex, this sensation of invisibility can be particularly debilitating. You become overly self-conscious, compulsively stealing peeks at mirrors, seeking reassurance that you are, in fact, still there, still beautiful, still desirable.

Even if you've never been a knockout, and, therefore, less accustomed to men jumping out of the woodwork, you still want to believe you're sexy to someone. You can rationalize that life is grand because your brain is spectacular, your career success has been stellar, your children are fabulously accomplished and your husband loves you just the way you are. However, unless diminishing hormones are causing you to lose all sexual interest, what you really want to be able to do is continue to inspire lust. Or, maybe that's just me. Hmmm. It seems idiotic, but I dread the day truckers stop honking at me.

At any rate, the minute a woman slips into this trough of insecurity, she cuts her sexual desirability in half. That goes for younger women, as well. When signs of age become far too visible — wrinkles, bubble butt, turkey neck — women begin to withdraw inside themselves. Some actually crouch in defeat, practically willing themselves to disappear.

My husband, who, bless his soul, actually prefers older women to younger ones, asked me why women had such issues with aging. I stumbled into an excellent explanation at a movie theater.

We were watching a preview in which Jack Nicholson's character recoiled in horror because he had accidentally stumbled into Diane Keaton's fifty-seven year old character naked. Jack went lurching out of the room with his hands over his eyes, hiding from the ultimate hideousness of middle-aged femininity saying, "Sorry, sorry, oh boy, am I sorry." Of course, there was no recoiling from the sight of his sixty year old ass in a hospital gown. It was merely comical and therefore cute.

"That," I said pointing a damning finger at the screen, "is the reason women have issues with aging." Then, I went on to say, "I'm boycotting this movie."

Of course, after I learned that Diane, smiling bravely and far too often, was the focus of Keanu Reeves' lust, not to mention Jack's (after he overcame his horror and decided that perky breasts weren't everything), I agreed to see it.

Diane might be one of six women in movies who hasn't had most of her parts cut off, lifted or replaced. The general rule from Hollywood is if you're past forty, or look like you're past forty, you're invisible as far as sexy leads are concerned. Hey, somebody's got to play grandma.

Speaking of grandma, that's who you'll be getting approached by as soon as you take the leap—or, should I say the fall—into fifty. You may think you look like you're thirty-five, but other women will set you straight in a heartbeat. You may actually have looked thirty-five when you were forty-nine but once you hit fifty you suddenly age fifteen years. It's like a cruel miracle.

Two years ago, my twenty-five year old niece told me I looked twenty-five. Last year, she told me I looked thirty. This year, I made the leap to forty, in her eyes. But, in the eyes of my peers, I'm a part of that sisterhood that has lots of turtlenecks in their wardrobes. What suddenly speeds the aging process to warp ten? The decline and fall of those goddamn hormones, that's what.

You can be standing on a grocery checkout line or changing in a locker room or vigorously hiking out of a volcanic crater when some old biddy with drooping cheeks and menopause red hair sidles over to you and ruins your day by assigning you to her age group. You'll feel like shouting, "Do I look fifty to you?" but instead you just smile through your pain at the poor delusional creature and talk about calcium supplements or retirement accounts or age spots.

As soon as you part company, you shoot a glance at yourself in a mirror to reassure yourself that you look decades younger than they, but the face that looks back at you doesn't give you that reassurance anymore. What can you do? For one thing, avoid side-view mirrors and fluorescent-lit dressing rooms with green walls. They actually do make you look fifty when you're twenty-five.

If you feel like you're disappearing at fifty, it's because you are. You're going through one of the biggest transitions of your life, beyond puberty. You know what you looked and felt like going in, but how are you going to look and feel when you emerge on the other side?

You may feel a sense of loss. You will have to mourn this loss and get on with your life in a new way. With the right attitude, you may be able to accomplish that without antidepressants, hormone supplements, liposuction or collagen injections. Maybe you'll begin a period of enlightenment in which you will realize that you are so much more than your face and body. That's what graceful aging is all about, and I will cover that toward the end of this book, after I've gotten a lot of bitching and moaning out of my system.

Always Something

❧

I went to an acupuncturist recently. She gave me drawings of a bemused-looking genderless naked person, front and back, and told me to make an X on corresponding parts of my body that hurt. By the time I was finished, I had completely crossed out both drawings. I was literally in pain from head to foot. The acupuncturist turned me into a porcupine.

It seems like you can freely abuse your body until the day before your fiftieth birthday. Beyond that, your body will be far less forgiving than you thought possible. Even if you've taken impeccable care of your body—as I have—fifty may still kick your ass—just because it can.

In the past year, I have heard the words, "Gee, I've never seen that before" emerge from too many doctors mouths. You end up with ailments you've never heard of, like subacute thyroiditis, which self-corrects if it doesn't kill you first.

One day, you're out enjoying some innocent activity, like kayaking, or maybe you're just sitting in a recliner working on a crossword puzzle, when your heart starts to race, you lose twelve pounds, your hair falls out and you start to hump floor lamps. A simple stroll from the bed to the bathroom makes you feel like *Dead Man Walking*, as you struggle for each breath. It can last for weeks.

What did I do to deserve this bizarre illness? Did I smoke cigarettes, drink bourbon, eat fast-food burgers, shoot heroin or have unprotected sex with unwashed strangers? No, I became a middle-aged woman and caught a mild case of the sniffles. That simple combo led me to the door of a life-threatening disorder. It sort of made me feel like going to the nearest bar and downing boilermakers with LSD chasers and making a porn flick with a kennel full of frisky Dobermans. What difference would it have made?

Of course, I get self-destructive thoughts every time I get a strange illness. In my thirties, it was a molar pregnancy. "What does that mean?" I asked my gynecologist. "Does the fetus have teeth?"

No, it was another one of those surprising, immensely rare life-threatening disorders. Aw shucks, what was the point in leading a healthy lifestyle? Actually, outside of the medical anomalies I've personally experienced, I think that living a healthy lifestyle makes a great deal of difference in the long run. It just won't stop weird shit from happening.

Middle-aged women have no monopoly on pain and misery. Middle-aged men get more than their share. In addition to big honcho afflictions like heart disease and cancer, they get nailed with enlarged prostates, gout, penile dysfunction and pesky nose hairs. But this is about women, so I'll let some man *kvetch* in his own book.

I wrote a few lyrics about the ailments of fifty-ish women. Sing this to the tune of *My Favorite Things*. (People are always putting words to this song that have nothing to do with whiskers on kittens.)

Migraine and eyestrain and neck pain and dry skin
Arthritis, bursitis, colitis and double chin
Bunions and reflux and dying to pee
That's what it's like to be turning fifty
　Flashes and bone loss and lots of depression
Insomnia, brain fog and other oppression
Weight gain and bleeding and feeling sleepy
That's what it's like to be turning fifty
　When the skin sags, when the breasts flop
When I'm feeling sad
I simply remember I'm fifty years old
And then I feel really bad

Every time you feel like things are going from bad to worse, remind yourself that things have never been that easy. Children, teenagers, young women and the aged certainly have their issues. Every period of life presents its own challenges and all that yakking about rolling with the punches is something to pay attention to. Nobody lives pain-free. You just have to learn how to manage it. Sometimes you have to make a few lifestyle changes. So what?

Eating right and exercising and maintaining a healthy weight and having great sex and being creative and having loving relationships and having a good attitude and inheriting the right genes may not be enough to keep you from getting dreadful illnesses, but they couldn't hurt. Make the most of what you've got through every stage of life. I figure if I play my cards right, I won't have to write a sequel to this book and call it *Kill Me Now, I'm Ninety.*

Medical Nightmares

⊰⊱

I'm not going to address the horrors of heart disease and cancer in this chapter. I'm merely going to bring up the routine tortures we're asked to endure just because we've made the mistake of slipping into middle age.

By the time you're forty, the AMA advises women to get mammograms once a year. By the time you're fifty, you actually know women who have breast cancer, so you make sure you keep your appointment, no matter how medieval it is.

When men ask me what a mammogram feels like, I tell them to imagine having their testicles compressed by a garage door and held in place for as long as it takes the technician to get the right grimace of pain on their face before she x-rays the aforementioned testicles, which now resemble undercooked pancakes.

For the past ten years, I've been held captive by a succession of mammogram technicians who report the statistics on breast cancer while I'm suspended by one squashed boob. There's no way to escape. All you can do is hang there and wait for the grim reaper to take the damn picture. If you're not scared when you go in there, you're certainly shaking in your shoes by the time you stagger out. You spend the next couple of weeks in fear that you will get a call, inviting you in for another look.

That actually happened to me once. Something looked suspicious on my x-ray, they said. After a sleepless night, I went flailing off to the hospital the next day and discovered about a hundred other women in the waiting room, all tensely awaiting their second look. We sat there in our blue smocks, wondering who would become a statistic that day. Some women had been there for hours, being called in for one test after another.

By the time my name was called, my voice was falsetto from fear. The tiny technician turned my breasts into corkscrews and lowered the garage door—I mean the compression device. I was too scared to feel any pain. I remarked on the number of women in the waiting room and asked her how often women received callbacks. "Oh honey, she said, "it happens all the time."

Her gentle words made me feel a little better, until she cranked my breast tissue down to the depth of toilet paper. "We want to get a real good picture this time," she said when she saw my eyes protruding from their sockets.

Once she released me and ran off with my new films, I put my blue smock back on and stood gazing at the anomaly on my earlier x-ray. I stared at the little glitch in my breast tissue and wondered if something that innocuous looking would be the beginning of the end for me. The technician came back a few minutes later and told me everything was fine, that my breast tissue had folded over onto itself during the previous mammogram—perhaps they had not compressed me enough. I collapsed on her in relief and tried not to look too thrilled when I passed the women who remained in the waiting room on my way out.

Another torture recommended for people, both women and men, past fifty is the colonoscopy, which requires you to purge yourself of everything you've ever eaten in your entire life so that a doctor may insert the equivalent of a garden hose into your rectum to go spelunking for polyps. At least they blast you into the twilight zone before they begin the procedure.

My dear husband loves colonoscopies for several reasons: one, he actually has the capacity to drink a gallon of Colyte; two, he enjoys spending hours on the toilet; and three, he loves the high he gets from the drugs involved. The prep lasts for hours. The procedure lasts ten minutes. The high lasts all day and, apparently, makes you horny, to boot.

My husband is probably alone in his enthusiasm for colonoscopies. The last time I had to purge for a test (not a colonoscopy, but another test that apparently required my intestines to be clean enough to eat out of), I was given the same prep kit as a three hundred pound man, and it nearly killed me. I may put a colonoscopy off until I'm sixty—at least. (Not that anyone else should do that—getting this test can save your life, so just disregard my silly-assed banter here.)

Let's get back into the exclusive realm of women. Almost every woman I know past the age of fifty has had a hysterectomy. Doctors have lots of reasons for yanking out uteri and ovaries. It usually has something to do with endometriosis or fibroids or excessive bleeding or a family history of cancer or the doctor's need to make a mortgage payment on his beach house.

If a woman is having "female troubles" and is finished with

childbearing, many doctors—predominantly male—will urge her to part with her "worthless" sex organs, thus launching her into surgical menopause instead of trying a less radical, non-surgical approach. Would a doctor suggest that a man have his testicles removed because he's impotent? Of course not! Would a doctor snip out a man's prostate gland because the man's father had prostate cancer? Get real.

Doctors, in general, seem to have a tremendous lack of regard for aging females' sex organs, not to mention the women they're housed in. When I was in my mid-forties and informed I was perimenopausal, I attended a seminar at a well-regarded women's hospital to learn more about it. The room was packed with women in different stages of menopause. They were all sitting there fanning themselves, waiting to be illuminated and comforted.

A male OB-GYN, who considered himself a menopause specialist, approached the podium with two sacks of nuts. One sack was chock full of big, perfect bright red pistachios. The other sack contained a mixture of deformed nuts and broken shells. He waved his big nut bag at us and said, "This is your sixteen-year-old daughter's ovaries." He then presented the bag of lame nuts and said, "And, these are your ovaries."

The room was silent. Did this idiot have a death wish? Maybe he was a *SOB*-GYN. Here we were, feeling lousy and terrified about losing our youthful femininity, and this flabby-assed "specialist" was confirming our worst fears. He was literally telling us we were becoming dried-up old hags. I personally felt like kicking him in his nut bags. Right or wrong, could you imagine the insensitivity?

Many women left. A few masochists, including myself, stuck around to hear the speech about the joys of hormone replacement therapy and how it would be the only way we could fend off heart disease, osteoporosis, dry skin, senility, hot flashes, brain fog, insomnia, vaginal atrophy, incontinence, hair loss, mood swings, tooth decay, St. Vitus dance and the heartbreak of psoriasis.

Okay, I added a few extra maladies, but I'm trying to emphasize the specialist's enthusiasm for synthetic hormones. That was shortly before HRT became hugely controversial and millions of women stopped taking it, preferring night sweats and shriveling vulvas to breast cancer, heart attacks and dementia.

Then, there are proponents of natural hormones. I was watching a program on public TV and the show featured an upbeat female internist who was addressing an audience of anxious-looking menopausal women, and, strangely enough, one man. The doctor gave these women (and one man) hope that if they did about a hundred different things a day (mostly having to do with giving up everything that makes life worth living and recording it all in a journal) on top of taking natural hormones, they would have a crack at a tolerable existence. Horribly enough, I agreed with nearly everything she said.

The doctor said, "Synthetic hormones, like Premarin, are made out of the urine of pregnant mares and that's not good for humans." (How many decades did it take for medical researchers to figure that one out?)

"Natural hormones, on the other, hand, are made from yams and soy, which are bio-identical to human hormones. Because they are bio-identical, there are fewer side effects." (What, there are fewer occurrences of spontaneous neighing?)

Huh? I'm no horse, but I yam not a soybean either! And what makes a yam or soybean more natural than horse urine? (All right, all right, the bio-identical angle—I may give it a shot. Desperate times call for desperate measures.)

All I can say about the whole matter is take the hormones if you must. There are herbal alternatives and supplements on the market that may help you out. Just keep in mind that they may be considered safe today and deadly tomorrow; who knows? Maybe the medical world will eventually come up with a bulletproof miracle for middle-aged women that will actually make us feel better rather than worse.

I would never advise you to disregard your doctor's orders, but don't be afraid to question them. Sometimes, doctors don't know squat about anything outside of their own specialty. For example, an ophthalmologist may not know that estrogen fluctuations can change the shape of the eye and be the first sign of menopause. Ophthalmologists know about eyes, and that's it. Gynecologists know about vaginas. They don't know or care about corneal abrasions. These specialists don't get the relationship between eyes and vaginas.

The truth is that every part of your body affects every other part. It's all connected. So, get to know your own body and try to make informed decisions about how to take care of it. You have a lot at stake.

Heal Yourself

❊

*T*he deeper you advance into middle age, the more things start to hurt. If you run to the doctor's office every time something hurts, you might as well rent a room there. By all means, go to the doctor for your routine exams and tests and take the medications they prescribe, provided the side effects don't have the potential to kill you.

Go to the doctor if you suspect you're having a stroke or heart attack. Go if you've been run over by your own car. Go if you feel a lump or have a weird-looking mole. Go if you're bleeding uncontrollably. Go if you have a flesh-eating staph infection.

I'm not saying don't go to the doctor. I'm just saying you can improve your chances of feeling tolerably well if you make a few, simple adjustments to keep the middle-aged monster at bay.

Most of the following suggestions are so obvious you're going to wonder why I'm mentioning them. I'll tell you why. People know what's good for them. They're just so addicted to what's bad for them, they would rather have a surgical procedure or take toxic drugs than change their habits.

For example, my friend, Louise, suffers from excruciating stomach pain and diarrhea after she's downed a couple of quarts of whole organic milk. Her doctors have told her that her age (forty-five) has made her increasingly lactose intolerant.

Louise confesses that she would rather be told she has gastrointestinal cancer than have to give up dairy products. Is this intelligent talk from a woman with a PhD from Stanford? Of course, not—but this talk has nothing to do with intelligence. It has to do with choices and what we're willing to sacrifice for our health and wellbeing. Here comes a practical list of do's and don'ts—and you've probably heard them before. Pay attention this time.

- If you're told you're lactose-intolerant, lay off the dairy. Find something else to satisfy your craving for cream—like soy products. Just don't gorge yourself. Too much of anything isn't good for you.
- If you have any other condition that requires you to restrict your diet, restrict your diet. It won't kill you.
- Drink as much water as you can stomach, including drinks that contain water, like tea. It'll keep your tissues hydrated and maybe keep you from looking like a catcher's mitt.
- As the yogis say, eat foods that are whole, fresh and pure. That means eat whole grains (even if they do have carbs), have plenty of fresh fruits and veggies, and avoid pesticides and additives like the plague. With a little luck, you won't find any locusts in your All Bran.
- In spite of what the yogis say, if you feel like having an

occasional hot fudge sundae with nuts and whipped cream, enjoy yourself, even if you are lactose intolerant. You've got to live a little. You may want to forget about the carcinogenic cherry on top.

- Some people swear by vitamins, minerals and herbs, including me. Some people think that vitamins, minerals and herbs only give you expensive urine and, occasionally, a blue tongue. Keep your own counsel.
- Don't deprive yourself of sunshine. You need the natural vitamin D to help you absorb calcium, and light helps you fight depression.
- Protect your skin if you're going to be out in the sun, especially if you're fair. Everybody looks better with a tan, until they're middle-aged. Then, they look like an alligator purse.
- Exercise as much as you can. Walk for heart health. Do yoga for flexibility and balance. Do Pilates for strength. Lift weights to ward off osteoporosis. Take the stairs to increase endurance. Swim to relieve arthritis. Dance for the pure joy of it.
- Don't smoke. It ages your skin, yellows your teeth, fouls your breath, damages your lungs and grosses me out.
- Form supportive relationships. You want to be around people who make you feel good about yourself. Try to avoid energy suckers, unless you don't mind having a one sided friendship.
- If your husband doesn't want to have sex with you, hire a pool boy—whether you have a pool or not. Being sexually active is important to your physical, spiritual, emotional and mental wellness.
- As you approach menopause, you will become less tolerant of stress and idiots. Try to avoid both.
- Keep a journal. It will help you objectify all the events of your

life and know yourself better. If you're afraid that someone will invade your privacy, tell him or her they sneak a peek at their own risk.

- Laugh more. Wrinkles turned upward are more attractive than wrinkles turned downward.

- If you're having trouble looking at yourself in the mirror, consider a facelift. Just be prepared to have to do it over and over again until you finally look like Michael Jackson — the most recent one.

- Maintain your creativity. Your energy level may flag, but don't allow yourself to plummet into mediocrity. Life is always worth living well.

- If you're a perfectionist, midlife is going to hit you like a sledgehammer. Try loving yourself more and cut yourself some slack. The skin on your throat probably looks crepier to you than it does to anyone else (except for the so-called friend who is actively willing you to get turkey neck before she does — and you don't need a friend like that).

Midlife Love

⚜

*L*ove can show up on your doorstep at any stage of life, and usually does when you least expect it. When it happens at midlife, you can sometimes have trouble believing it's really happening because by the time you're fifty, you've got baggage. You may even look like baggage. But, no matter how insecure you may feel, take heart, you're not alone. Venturing into the love arena makes everybody feel insecure, but it's worth the trip. Finding romantic love at midlife can make the back fifty feel great—better than a bathtub full of chocolate.

How likely is it that you will find true love at fifty? If you're satisfied with your life as is, then it's likely you've already found it. If you're wandering around feeling like the living dead, you're probably more receptive to connecting with someone. Midlife is a time of change and it often provides us with opportunities to start anew, if we have the courage and desire do so and don't allow ourselves to get hung up in a web of inertia.

What has your relationship scenario been so far and how willing are you to change in order to find someone different? Is different necessarily better or are you merely exchanging one set of baggage for another? Is happiness just an illusion, as the song goes, or is it an attainable goal?

Here is a story I hear over and over again:

I've been with my husband for more than twenty years. I married him because it seemed like the right thing to do at the time. I wanted to have kids and a comfortable home life and my husband had all the right credentials—similar background, good family and a promising future. I think I loved him, maybe. If I didn't, I figured I would learn to over the years. Then, real life happened, along with real children and mortgage payments, and I began to resent him because I never did learn to love the SOB. Now, I feel like he's a stranger in my bed, and not one I want to sleep with. We don't seem to have anything in common, except for the kids, and they're going to be out of the house soon. We're either fighting or avoiding each other. We tried counseling, but my heart wasn't in it. I'd like to ditch him altogether, but then what? Will I have enough to live on? Where will the kids go for Christmas? What will our friends and family say? What am I going to do, move into a studio apartment? I'm almost fifty, who's going to want me? I think I'll go to the spa and get a manicure.

Here's another one:

I love my wife. Really. We have a terrific life together—nice home, great kids, and a house in the country. We're active in our church and community. We have plenty of money. We ski and cruise and play tennis. Did I say we have great kids? Our life is very well organized, like a business. Did I say I love my wife? We enjoy getting together with friends and taking family vacations. We don't have a big romance going on and we haven't had sex in fifteen years, but, hey, we're a good team. I don't want to divorce my wife—after all, our life is almost perfect. So, what am I supposed to do? Accept celibacy at fifty? Fall in love with my left hand? Become a hound from hell and sleep with as many women as possible, including prostitutes? Have a secret romance with one special woman? Do you want to go to Amsterdam with me this weekend?

What do these two people have in common, aside from the fact they're both screaming? Quite a lot, actually—maybe they should pair up.

She (I'll call her Amy) went into her marriage with an agenda the length of the *Magna Charta*. Hers was a marriage of practicality—a means to an end. Amy would never be able to love her husband in a fulfilling way. Yet, there are aspects of her life that work, so she rationalizes keeping her marriage intact, as long as she can disengage from it and avoid real intimacy with her husband (I'll call him Joe Schmo). She probably daydreams about having an affair with the white knight, provided he agrees not to wear his helmet in bed.

I'm going to call the guy in the second scenario Joe Schmo because—surprise!—he's Amy's clueless husband.

Joe thinks he's got it all and truly believes he's been the ideal husband. He's been supportive of her career, provided for his children and given his family everything money can buy. All he wants to do is work hard, play a little golf on weekends, maybe buy a vintage roadster and get a little love at home. Unfortunately, the only time Amy allows him to touch her is out in public, to demonstrate to the world how happy they are. Joe misses the boat when he goes along with this pretense and doesn't press for more behind closed doors. He's afraid to ask for what he wants because he knows in his heart that his wife has never loved him. He distracts himself with mindless porn, instead.

What's sad about this all-too-common situation is that Amy and Joe may have thought they loved each other at the beginning, while family and friends were influencing them. But, community and tradition would only support them so far. Ultimately, they had to face each other without an audience and that's when they saw a stranger's eyes looking back.

Can this marriage be saved? Not in any enjoyable way. Amy will always be angry with Joe because he's not the man of her dreams. And Joe will always be insecure because he'll be forced to live with Amy's unrelenting ire. This couple was doomed from the start because there was no foundation of true love to begin with. They've led a smoke-and-mirrors life.

If Amy continues to live her life with a grocery list of expectations, she can probably kiss off any hope of true love with anyone. If Joe doesn't start to express his desires, he will probably become a hound from hell in his attempt to overcome his loneliness, not to mention his suppressed canine lust.

If there is a second or third or fourth time around for this couple, maybe they will learn that love has nothing to do with power, ulterior motive or what other people think. In the end, it's just the two of them and they have to be able to look at one another without cringing or rolling their eyes.

On the other hand, most people don't live in a vacuum. Life is larger than a couple in a room, unless you're talking about an affair and that's a whole other chapter. In the world of "real" relationships, if you live with anybody long enough, they're bound to get on your nerves. Before you make the ultimate decision to flee, you must first learn to distinguish between occasional nettling and perpetual misery. One can be handled with an afternoon of shopping and a romantic matinee. The other may require more drastic measures — like separate bedrooms, at least.

The Affair—A Whole Other Chapter

*M*y old friend, Barry, is an advocate for polygamy. Twenty years ago, he and his wife vowed to love, honor and sleep with as many people as possible, with each other's permission and encouragement. Yikes.

Barry claims that he and his wife, Laura, have a great marriage, are in love with each other and enjoy a very satisfying sex life; that is, when Laura isn't off in Paris or Los Angeles or Calgary enjoying romances with various boyfriends. Everybody wants a piece of Laura. Barry is delighted for her, but doesn't quite get why he's not outscoring his wife.

"Getting any?" I ask Barry.

"Well, no, actually, I'm not," he says.

"Why do you suppose that is?" I ask.

"I don't know," he says, truly clueless. "I'm very honest with everyone. When I see a woman I'm attracted to, I tell her I'm married and in love with my wife, but would like to have a no-strings-attached sexual relationship. I even tell them it's okay with my wife."

"Are you approaching married women?"

"Well, no. I don't want somebody's husband punching me in the mouth."

"So, let me get this straight. You're approaching single women and telling them you want to screw them without possibility of a real relationship? What is their reaction?"

"Well, they sort of back out of the room and I never see them again."

"Who are you, Johnny Wad? You're a hairy dentist from Secaucus. Of course, they're backing away."

Barry still doesn't get it.

For the sake of this chapter, a "real" relationship is one in which you can have dinner together in public without Groucho masks, make out in a movie theater with impunity and watch TV together in your underwear, with the lights on and the shades open.

Typically, men will have sex with any willing woman, even if she's a hairy female dentist from Secaucus. Single women, on the other hand, are usually looking for real relationships — not one-night stands with married dentists. Okay, the selfish bitch from chapter two may sleep with your husband, but she's an exception.

Married women are another story. More and more, they are stepping out and having affairs. Some are in it for the sex. Take my friend, Kay, for example.

Kay is a fabulously successful, hot-looking woman at the tail end of forty-nine. All three of her children are randy teenagers, trawling the Internet for porn and attending oral sex parties. Kay is roasting in a vat of raging hormones. Unfortunately, her husband can't (or doesn't want to) get it up. She's decided that when she turns fifty, she's going to celebrate by finding a guy that can satisfy her strong sexual desires with no strings attached.

Maybe I should give her Barry's number. They even live in the same state!

Unlike Kay, most women have affairs out of sheer loneliness. No matter how long they've been with their spouses, they're just not getting the attention they need. Either their husbands travel for business, or they're obsessing over work, or they're hanging out with the boys or they're in a twelve-step program.

The couple may raise children, handle family business and run a household together but they talk about nothing else and rarely touch. Every once in a while he slips it to her for a few minutes in the dark before passing out. If the woman tells her husband she needs more and he doesn't hear her — or doesn't care — then her marriage is a divorce — or an affair — waiting to happen. All she needs to do is meet the right man — hopefully someone who can offer her more than her husband or Barry. She's missing a lot more than sex.

The difference between a divorce and an affair depends upon the woman's confidence level, how independent she is and the extent of her need. Kay has everything but sex. She just wants to get laid. The lonely woman has everything but love, baby. She has the most to gain and the most to lose from an affair. She wants a relationship but unless she's ready to go the distance, an affair is going to be unlike any real relationship she's ever had.

Here's another affair in the making: twenty years worth of routine sex. If you find yourself thinking, "We're screwing, it must be seven in the morning on Tuesday," you know you're about to be bored into illicit action, if you haven't already lost your interest in sex entirely. If you find yourself just lying there and taking it like it's medicine or making valiant attempts to get your partner off in a hurry so you can get on with your day, you either have to shake things up with your partner or come up with an alternative means of satisfying yourself—that is, if it is, in fact, important to you. I hope it's important to you. You're fifty; you're not dead.

I am not saying that a divorce or affairs are the only two options for lonely, bored or sexually deprived women—or men, for that matter. People sublimate their needs all the time and in all sorts of ways. They throw themselves into career, into children, into gardening, into yoga, into religion, into book clubs, into investing, into travel—the list goes on and on. And then there's marital counseling.

Couples go into counseling even when they know there's no bringing back that loving feeling *'cause it's gone, gone, gone.* At the risk of upsetting lots of people, I'll bet that affairs save more marriages than counseling—if both participants go into it with the right attitude (i.e., no demands and no expectations), both want the same thing, and both have a proper consideration for their spouses. It's avoidance, all right, but it does take the pressure off the conflicted couple.

"Don't want to talk to me? Not a problem—I'll talk to someone else. Don't find me sexually appealing. No problem—someone else will. Want to spend another week at the hunting lodge, sweetie? That's okay. I'll call Carlo and have the pool cleaned."

You get my drift.

Affairs are complicated. A few couples overtly give each other permission to have outside relationships—ala Barry and Laura. In some relationships, permission is more tacit. Either one partner or the other is getting what they need from the marriage but are not interested in or unable to engage sexually with their mate—ala Kay and her husband. So, they give each other a silent nod, look away, trust their partner to be discrete and continue to live their lives.

Most often, affairs are secret and, therefore, dangerous business. Discovery almost always results in jealous rage, hurt feelings and the occasional onsite castration. People don't do well with surprises like that. But, some women are so desperate for their husband's attention, they will engage in an affair and actually court detection just to get a rise out of their spouse.

If everybody survives and there is deep feeling left between husband and wife, the marriage may get back on track if both partners put in a huge effort, with or without the aid of a counselor…except if a pregnancy occurs. That can be a showstopper unless the husband is very, very understanding.

Don't mistake perimenopause for infertility. That's where change-of-life babies come from. You may have nothing to fear from your neutered husband, but if you're having unprotected sex with an unfixed partner, you can end up having a lot of *'splainin'* to do.

Sometimes, whether you're single or married, horny or lonely, you just fall in love and all reason goes right out the window. You start to feel young and beautiful and carefree in your lover's arms. He's so charming and passionate. But then, while you're donning your Groucho mask for a rare dinner out with the heavily-baggaged man of your dreams, he calls and tells you that he won't be able to make it—he and his wife of thirty years are taking off for the country with their three children and two dogs (Bonzo and Lambchop) and throwing a big party for family and friends, not including you. Is your life really worth this trade-off?

Get real.

But sometimes—just sometimes—you end up in a better place. The miracle of soul mating does happen and a far more fulfilling union can occur. Don't talk yourself out of taking a chance with someone new and give up on the possibility of a better relationship — he may be your last chance at the golden ring. If your feelings are mutual, sometimes you've just got to close your eyes and jump. The rest of the people in your life will have to adjust.

Left In The Middle

❀

*D*ivorce is traumatic at any age. When you're left at midlife, it can be downright deadly, especially if you're left for someone with functioning ovaries (her day will come, don't worry about it).

When a marriage hasn't worked in years and children are finally grown and out of the house, some women may choose to dissolve their marriage, especially if they are financially independent and already involved with another man. Women of fifty don't typically move on without a safety net, unless their husbands are mean, abusive drunks or worthless deadbeats. Even then, most women stick around. It's amazing how much crap we'll take, especially when our self-image takes a nosedive into hell during midlife.

Middle-aged men have a whole litany of reasons for seeking divorce: too much nagging; too little sex; too many tantrums; too little understanding of their needs; too many arguments about money; too little support for their ambitions; too much pressure; too little time left to waste one more minute on a loveless, energy-draining, ball-breaking union that should've ended years ago but didn't. Oh, and the other woman's ass is firmer than yours.

Whatever the reason, when a man announces that he's leaving, the woman is almost invariably devastated...even if she initiated the separation.

"Where do you think you're going?" she wails.

"You threw me out, remember?"

"I didn't mean it. Will you pick up a quart of milk on your way home?"

"I'm not coming home this time."

"What do you mean, you're not coming home. Don't you know I love you, you limp-dicked, worthless fucking asshole?"

You get the gorgeous picture. Of course, in this case, your sympathies may be with the man, and with good reason. I know of several cases in which I have admired the man's intestinal fortitude for sticking around with a shrill, soul-shattering wife. On the other hand, I could present another scenario or two that would make you want to run out and buy a polo mallet. In fact, I think I will.

A strange man approached me in the library, where I sat in a quiet corner working on this very book, and he decided that what he had to say was more important than what I had to write. I told him I had work to do, but he was undeterred and actually seemed desperate to talk. I agreed to give him twenty minutes of my time and ended up listening to him for three hours. Then, I cut him off— but not before he had given me valuable insight into the workings of the middle-aged man's mind, especially as it related to middle-aged women.

He was a nice looking pilot in his early forties. He'd been married three times, each time to an older woman. His current wife was fifty and dying of cancer. They had two small children. He told me that his wife was bossy and disrespectful. He used that as an excuse to justify hitting her and throwing her out of the house. He claims he wanted out before he knew she had cancer. Oh, and he couldn't wait to marry his twenty-one year old French girlfriend. He was particularly miffed that his wife hadn't signed the divorce papers yet (maybe she was too busy getting chemo treatments and taking care of two children under the age of five while she was dying alone and recovering from being hurled into the street). He couldn't understand why her family treated him like a war criminal.

Okay, I'm glad I purchased the polo mallet.

Here's another story. Joe and Jeanette had been married for thirty years. They had two grown daughters. Joe had a lucrative position with an insurance company and Jeanette was a former runway model. Joe wanted to drop out of the corporate world and become a fashionably starving artist. Jeanette had chronic fatigue syndrome and a tendency to nap a lot, sometimes mid-sentence. Joe said he still loved Jeanette but he was no longer in love with her — after thirty years, the passion had ebbed — and he was disturbed that Jeanette was unsupportive of his need to express himself creatively, so he filed for divorce.

So desperate was he for escape, he gave Jeanette all his assets and moved three states over. It still took Jeanette seven years to sign the divorce papers.

Today, Joe is finally free to starve alone, and he's never been happier. Past sixty, he wears a ponytail and tank tops and pops Viagra. Younger women are happy to take him in because they find his free spirit sexy. In the meantime, Jeanette is down and out in Delaware. The money she received from Joe has been small solace. She hooked up with the first man who was willing to be her caretaker. She is now living as his thrall, forbidden to make the simplest decisions for herself. Desperation has turned her into a prisoner. She shares her misery with her daughters but they're trying to live their own lives. They love her but are relieved that she is in some else's care, no matter how restrictive.

I admit, middle-aged women can be a handful. Nevertheless, some men have the maturity or love or family values or whatever it takes to hang in there while their partners go through what is probably the most difficult years of their lives. These men are actually honoring the vows they made on their wedding day, when they promised to stick around for better or for worse. A woman's passage into midlife is usually for worse, at least temporarily. A loving mate can make the transition much easier for her, but a lot of men can't handle the responsibility of caring for a dysfunctional spouse…especially one who won't give them any.

On the other hand, middle-aged men are going through their own crises. Their friends are keeling over left and right from heart attacks and strokes. They may be losing out to younger men and women in the job market. They may be losing their hair, their sexual potency and the ability to see their own feet beneath their bellies. Even their golf swing may be off. If they're afraid they are failing and their wives reinforce this fear, they may fall into their own hopeless despair. They may feel driven to escape and try to resurrect their lives.

Men may struggle with their decision to leave but once their minds are made up, they get out in a hurry, at all cost, with a deep sigh of relief. Women, on the other hand, may be miserable in their marriages, but, even if their husbands have behaved abominably, they still hold onto them like grim death.

Part of that clinging behavior is punitive in nature. Jilted wives need to make their husbands suffer for leaving them. Refusing to sign divorce papers or milking their fleeing husbands for all their worth gives them a small, smug but ultimately empty sensation of power. Most women hold on because they are terrified of being alone. Their fantasy of growing old with men they shared their lives with is shot to hell and they lack the strength or desire to start over.

For those women who have been left at midlife, I urge you to do whatever you can to regain your self-esteem and achieve independence. Get back to work. Go back to school. Join a support group. Do volunteer work. Speak with a counselor. Get into shape. Take a trip. Lose your agendas. Beware of men who prey on desperate, lonely women, especially if you have financial assets. And, don't give up hope on falling in love again. You may end up happy beyond your wildest dreams once you truly cut the cord on your previous life.

Changing Careers

·=·×·×·=·

*W*hen we're in our twenties and fresh out of school, we can't wait to put our degrees to work. Most of us are footloose with few responsibilities aside from paying off school loans and making sure our deadbeat roommates contribute their share of the rent. We've got more energy than a bag full of squirrels.

We land entry-level positions at corporations, eager to please our bosses. We're willing to work eighty hours a week for relatively meager pay, just so we can get promoted to the next level where we will work a hundred hours a week for a little more. We leap into airplanes at the drop of a hat with all kinds of electronic devices dangling from our bodies and keep a packed bag ready at the front door.

Or, maybe we're highly-driven young doctors or mothers or teachers or journalists, all on a quest to be the best in our field, earn the most, achieve the highest honors, raise the next Sally Ride, make the biggest difference in the world. Some of us are just motivated to get our own apartment. Whatever, we're at a highly jazzed stage of life. We're at the beginning of the big adventure that is our life.

At my tenth high school reunion, all anyone wanted to talk about were careers, and for good reason. Up until this time, most of our lives were spent getting educated and trained for what we were going to be when we grew up. An accomplished person of twenty-eight is justifiably proud of his or her achievement. Business cards sporting impressive titles are passed out like jellybeans at an Easter picnic.

At the twentieth reunion, the conversation shifts to family. People are brandishing pictures of their spouses and children, bragging of their accomplishments. Career is still very important — in fact, at this point we're probably at the top of our game — but typically, it's not just about us anymore. All that travel is getting old. We don't look as good in those terrible khaki pants and golf shirts they make almost everybody wear at trade shows. We miss seeing our children grow up.

By the time we get to the thirtieth reunion, most of us have experienced some kind of loss — of a parent, of a spouse, of a career, of our health — and we start to reevaluate what's important to us. Life has buffeted us about a bit and has hopefully made us richer, fuller, more complex and more compassionate, maybe less self-involved. Instead of trying to see ourselves through others' eyes, we are more willing to see them.

There's a wonderful change afoot. Some of us are realizing that there's more to us than meets the eye (which is a good thing because some of us aren't looking that hot anymore). We're on the verge of exploring what else life has to offer, starting anew with a different set of goals. We've had the big career, we've had the fifty thousand dollar wedding (or two or three), we've had the kids (or not), we've proven ourselves in one way or the other, and we've had some big wins and some big losses. We've survived. Now, we want to live.

Many alumni will not show up to their fortieth reunion because they'll feel like mere shadows of their former selves. The ones that do come may yank out pictures of grandchildren and vacation homes, but they'll feel downsized almost out of existence unless they're continuing to lead a productive, if not gainful, life. The individuals who have given up on life are the folks that dwell on the downside of aging and regale you with stories about their gall bladder operations, liposuction surgery and cravings for Metamucil milkshakes, while they're having a senior moment and forgetting your name.

A lot of women feel deeply diminished when their careers or motherhood wind down. It's not necessarily because they miss the work, the travel, the stress and the aggravation — they just have the awful feeling that life will lose all meaning when they no longer bear an impressive title like CEO or MOM.

If you absolutely love the work you've been doing for the past twenty-five years and need the money and prestige, I say, by all means, stick with it. If you still have kids at home at age fifty, you have my condolences. If you have achieved financial independence by midlife and have the chance to do whatever your heart desires, congratulations, may you take advantage of this great opportunity.

The problem is, lots of women don't recognize this freedom as an opportunity. They see it as a fall from grace, something to be ashamed of or guilty about.

I recently sat next to a middle-aged stranger at a dinner party who whispered in my ear behind a cupped hand that she had left her high-powered career as an advertising executive in a large corporation to make fudge at a candy store for minimum wage. She was having a ball but her wealthy, retired husband was aghast. The thought of his wife publicly cramming almonds into chocolates for peanuts was almost more than he could bear. I thought it was great that she was being creative and enjoying herself at the same time and sorry that her husband was such a tight ass. I told her my husband wouldn't mind if I took up table dancing, as long as it made me happy. She and I had a private chuckle together. Her husband would have requested a separate table if he heard us.

When I attend my fortieth reunion, I want to be able to say that my life truly started anew at fifty. The only way I'm going to be able to say that is by putting my money where my mouth is. If I've been in marketing for twenty-five years and want to become a screenplay writer, I won't give up my day job (unless I'm financially independent, and who is?) but I will also start to write plays, take classes and take the steps necessary to realize my dream. If I'm tired of being a lawyer (and who isn't?), I may train to become a yoga instructor. You get my drift.

The message here is simple: Don't be afraid of changing careers midstream. Midlife crisis can be a good thing. It makes us aware of what's not working in our lives and, unless we allow it to defeat us, it can propel us onto a far more satisfying and balanced path. If you want to run like a racehorse forever, you may as well be on the right track. Find out what you love to do and do it, with no apologies to spouses, children or strangers at dinner parties. Creativity (and maybe a little moisturizer) helps keep you young.

By the way, if you're looking for a job in the corporate world and you're a woman past fifty, your chances of landing a position are extremely diminished; I don't care what anyone says. Ageism and sexism are, in fact, alive and well in corporate America.

You can look like you're thirty, but if you've had more than twenty-five years worth of experience, you might as well accept that the twenty-eight-year-old with three years worth of experience you're competing with is probably going to get the job. Sure, she may need to go on maternity leave at some point, but she will probably require a much lower salary, work twice as hard, not have to fan herself at meetings and not be as likely to challenge the boss, who's probably thirty-five. Think about it.

Start your own business and you won't have to deal with this kind of discrimination - especially if you telecommute and never leave your basement office.

The Midlife Workout

⚜

When I turned fifty, I insisted on getting a bone scan, just for grins. I figured, hey, I take calcium with magnesium and vitamin D, I exercise, I eat broccoli several times a week, I don't smoke or drink, I still get periods and my mother's solid as a rock. I expected to have the bone density of a tyrannosaurus rex. Turns out, I had the bone mass of a boiled chicken.

The scan revealed that I was working my way toward osteopenia. I had never heard of osteopenia. I asked my doctor if it meant I was growing a dick. Only kidding. Actually, I asked him if I had unusually low bone mass for a woman my age that was not on hormone replacement therapy. He quickly assured me that my bone loss was quite usual and that we all start to lose bone mass at around thirty. As a slim person, I started out with slender bones to begin with so I had less to lose before I qualified as low normal—lucky little me.

Actually, I am lucky. My doctor told me to ratchet up my calcium intake to fifteen hundred milligrams a day and get more weight bearing exercise. There would be no need for nauseating bone-building meds — yet. I was off the next day to look for a health club.

It's important to find a club you feel at home in or you'll never go. If you don't have children, you're not going to want to join a family-oriented health club unless you don't mind ingesting baby urine and having kids jump on your head in the pool. You probably don't want to join a club that has a boxing ring at the front door or a steroid concession in the basement. And, you need to find a club with reasonable temperature control or you may get a terminal case of hot flashes and drown in your own sweat, mid-crunch. It could happen.

I managed to find a fabulous club about four miles from my house, with lots of branches within a reasonable distance if I wanted a change of scenery. The club is big and bright and cool, with lots of beautifully maintained workout equipment and free weights, along with a pool, basketball court, hot tub, sauna, showers — the works.

The thing I love most about my club is that it offers a pile of courses that are included in the cost of membership. In addition to fiddling with weights and swimming laps, I take yoga twice a week, Pilates twice a week and something called Latin Impact, which is an hour's worth of salsa and swing dancing without a partner. I've seen women of twenty crawling out of that one after fifteen minutes. (Heh heh heh.)

My only complaint about the club is that aggressive personal trainers try to convince you you're in terrible shape so they can sell you their services.

I got set up with a young Nazi named Duke who asked me,

"What would you say if I told you that you could look your best at one fifty?"

I'm five foot six and weigh about one hundred and twenty pounds, mostly muscle.

"Duke," I said, "I have no desire to look like Xena the Warrior Princess' mother."

Duke rose to the challenge and took another approach. He told me I had a body mass index of twenty-seven (it's actually nineteen, but whose counting) and said "our" goal was to get it down to fourteen.

"Duke," I said, "I have no desire to look like a prepubescent boy from Biafra."

I could tell I was pissing Duke off, but he was about to make me pay for it. He put me through a workout that disabled me for three days. My thighs were so stiff I had to go to the bathroom standing up. I didn't sign up for additional sessions.

The club tried again. This time, I was set up with a young woman named Leslie who had red braids, a weight problem and an angry disposition. She looked at me and said, "You should weigh thirty pounds more." I was about to say, "You should weigh sixty pounds less," but I remembered my disabling experience with young Duke and decided to zip it. This one looked like she could stuff me through a basketball hoop.

"Only free weights build bone mass," said Leslie, the Amazon Queen. "The weight machines are for the sick and the weak."

I took a gander at the gorillas on the weight machines and they didn't look like they were ailing to me. Still, I was willing to believe that free weights offered a more effective workout. I was anxious to hear more.

Leslie showed me a thing or two and told me that if I wanted to see more, I'd have to buy a package of sessions. My husband had bought a few sessions with Leslie. She showed him a thing or two for about ten minutes, and then sent him to the treadmills. That way, his sessions ended up costing him about eighty dollars a minute. Nice work, if you can get it.

I decided I had seen enough…especially after I saw a grandma in pastel pink warm-ups pumping away in the weight room, working her way toward a BMI of nine, presumably before she disappeared completely.

What is a reasonable workout for middle-aged women? It's best to consider what you're trying to accomplish and use a little common sense. We all want to keep our weight under control. We're all trying to build, or at least preserve, bone mass. We want well-toned muscles. We want to exercise our hearts. We want to increase flexibility. We all want more energy. And, we want to relieve stress.

All of this can be accomplished without joining a gym, of course. If you eat sensibly, drink water and take a swift walk in the fresh air a few times a week, you will likely lose weight, exercise your heart and feel energized at the same time.

Personally, I much prefer a walk in the woods to a walk on a treadmill because I enjoy the experience of actually going somewhere when I move. Of course, if you're on a treadmill, you probably don't have to run from the occasional yellow jacket. (The best aerobic exercise I ever got was fleeing from an angry swarm while cursing at the top of my lungs. My husband told me I actually leaped over a ravine, but I don't remember. I was too busy screaming.)

To build bone and muscle mass, buy a couple of three or five pound weights and lift them a few times a week. You may even want to swing them while you walk. Just be aware of who's around you so you don't knock anybody's teeth out.

For flexibility and balance, try yoga. For strength, do Pilates, if you can do them without rupturing your pelvis. You can buy videos and do the exercises at home or take classes. If you take a class, go at your own pace. These are not competitive sports. With the right spirit, you may very well enjoy the chemistry of the group and you get to wear cute outfits. At least, the instructor gets to wear cute outfits — he or she has been practicing for a while and can really pull off Spandex.

It's never too late to start a tai chi program. In fact, the older you are, the better because tai chi requires patience. It's great for flexibility and balance, both physical and emotional, and looks really cool when you synchronize with a group and do it on a hillside.

Dancing is great exercise. It gets your heart pumping and tones your whole body. Do it with or without a partner. Yes, you can dust and boogie at the same time.

Speaking of doing it with or without a partner, make sure you integrate sex into your workout schedule. It's probably the best exercise you can get. Get those endorphins flowing with a little Dr. Love. No equipment is required, but it's available if you want it.

Before you begin a fitness program, make sure you consider your own personal condition and health issues. When you first start to work out, you may feel a little stiff for a few days. (Thanks, Duke.) That's to be expected. There may be exercises you shouldn't be doing.

Don't do anything that hurts. If you're experiencing pain, stop. If you're menopausal, you probably already feel lousy. Maybe you should let somebody else feel the burn. You don't have to kill yourself to get into shape, although sometimes it may feel that way.

Do what you enjoy. Do what makes sense for you. If you're not having any fun, you'll end up on the couch eating bonbons. Set realistic goals and you will see results.

What Shall I Eat?

~❧~

*E*at protein. Eliminate carbs. Stay away from refined sugar. Tote that barge and lift that bale. For the love of Mike, use your head. If you're approaching fifty, you already know if you have a weight problem or not. If you do, midlife is not going to help your case because, typically, our metabolisms slow down and we can't be as self-indulgent as we once were without paying the price: becoming a lard bucket.

Some of us are built to carry a little extra weight. How are (or were) your parents built? If you have a hefty parent to take after — or, worse yet, two — weight control is going to be more of a challenge. You do inherit a body type. However, you do not have to inherit a propensity to overeat. The old saw about moderation makes sense.

Barring certain steroids and antidepressants, medical conditions such as hypothyroidism, genetic predispositions or psychological stumbling blocks, losing weight and keeping it off is largely a function of eating sensibly, exercising regularly and drinking plenty of water. Period. There's no need to knock yourself out of balance with extreme diets or exercise regimens, which are hard to maintain at best and deadly at worst.

The worst thing you can do if you're trying to lose weight is to deny yourself. If you feel deprived, I can guarantee you that you will end up eating more. You may sneak it when nobody's looking, but you're only fooling yourself. You've got to know that that secret cheesecake is going to show up on your hips. That's going to depress you even more, which means you will soon be having a midnight date with an economy-sized bag of peanut buttercups.

Lots of us are in a state of denial over why we are overweight. We may say, "I don't understand why I'm gaining so much weight. I'm hardly eating anything." We forget about the pans of brownies we devour after midnight when nobody's looking.

Who are we trying to kid?

Bad eating habits begin in childhood. They're hard to break, but, if you want to be a healthy adult, you're going to have to make a few adjustments.

Busy life styles may make it difficult to eat healthfully. A rushed existence lends itself to too many fast food meals on the run, too many prepared foods, too many hi-cal restaurant meals. By the time you reach midlife, let's hope that things have slowed down for you a little so you can eat in peace.

Here are a few basic suggestions for eating well and keeping weight from gaining on you:

- Eat as many fruits and vegetables as you want.
- Drink as much water as you can stand.
- Minimize or eliminate red meat from your diet. If you do crave meat, trim the fat first.

- Minimize your intake of bread, potatoes, pasta, fried foods, processed foods, refined sugar, sodium and desserts.
- Eat more fish and lean poultry. Avoid chicken skin.
- Eat whole grains like buckwheat, oats and brown rice.
- Sprinkle a couple of tablespoons of ground flaxseed on your whole grain cereal—it'll lower your cholesterol and keep you regular.
- Eat slowly, savoring each bite.
- Minimize or eliminate soft drinks and alcohol.
- Minimize or eliminate whole milk dairy products.
- Try not to eat within three hours of going to bed. If you must have a snack (I know I do), try unbuttered popcorn popped in olive oil, roasted soybeans or a handful of raw almonds.
- Drink one to two cups of green tea a day.
- Avoid weight-loss supplements, especially those containing ephedra—unless you think that death is a good weight-loss strategy.
- Allow yourself the occasional indulgence—anything you want. Just don't eat enough to overstuff a water buffalo.
- Keep moving. Barring medical conditions that preclude it, there's nothing better for you than a swift walk in the fresh air. Here's the eating part: Do not chew while in motion.
- Fall in love. It's better than chocolate.

If you're already doing all this (really) and you're not losing weight, get your thyroid checked or find out if one of your ancestors was in the circus. If you just can't lose the weight, don't be too hard on yourself. There's nothing wrong with a few curves, as long as you're healthy and feel good.

The Middle-Aged Image

⁂

Twenty years ago, when I was still working in the corporate world, my friend, Sandra, asked me if I would ghost write a book for her on the subject of professional image. Back then, the typical business attire for women consisted of a gray or navy suit with a knee-length skirt or straight-legged pants, a silk blouse with a neck bow, taupe nylons and black medium-height pumps. Hair was to be kept on the short side and neatly coifed.

I sat across the table from Sandra in my peasant dress and high-heeled sandals, my gypsy hair flowing wildly down my back and started to laugh.

"You want me to tell other women how to dress for success in corporate America armed only with gray or navy gabardine? Look at me! I dress like a flamenco dancer!"

I didn't end up working on the book, which is unfortunate because it was quite successful. It was chock full of people dressed like they were attending a Baptist convention—very conservative, very clean, very uniform, very appropriate, very *Stepford Wives*. Not that there's anything wrong with that.

I was hardly ever appropriate, but that never kept me out of the boardroom. Maybe I was given a little more rope because I was a marketeer and therefore considered a creative type. Whatever. I was always a nonconformist when it came to uniformity and regimentation. (I got thrown out of the Brownies when I was six for refusing to wear the beanie and ankle socks. And, I would probably get thrown out of the Red Hat Society for the same reason. You may want to keep that in mind as you read this chapter.)

I'm a bit unconventional when it comes to fashion—but I promise I won't tell you to wear a red hat (unless you are also wearing a red garter). I'm going to tell you to wear whatever makes you feel good and look fantastic; not like an escapee from *Monty Python*.

Many people don't really know what their bodies look like and their clothing reflects their unawareness. I don't mean they don't know if they're fat or skinny. I mean they haven't seen themselves from every angle and, therefore, do not know how to make the most of their assets.

Here are a few personal observations for mid-lifers. Hardly anybody's butt looks good in khaki pants. Nobody looks good in Bermuda shorts. Turtlenecks may cover turkey necks, but they will also call attention to your jowls. If you're carrying a few extra pounds, you may want to avoid Spandex and thongs. And, the old hooker look is definitely out, unless you're at a costume party—or unless you actually are an old hooker.

Dressing comfortably is very important, especially if you are suffering from hot flashes. Wear natural fabrics that breathe and layer your apparel, so you can easily accommodate your body's fluctuating temperatures.

Don't be afraid of color. In fact, revel in color. Find out which hues work with your complexion and hair shade and have a ball bringing out your beautiful eyes and your sensuous lips, or what have you. Of course, there's no need to look like a circus clown. For a subtler look, splashes of color work just fine.

Basic black works for just about everybody, but there's no need to look like a widow from the old country. That's where accessories come in — soft pashminas, elegant jewelry, silk scarves. If you have an hourglass figure, show it off with belts and sashes. Lay off the fishnets.

If you happen to have a fantastic body, feel free to wear belly shirts and short shorts — just don't wear them in front of your teenaged daughter's boyfriend. It's important to dress appropriately — you don't want to wear a fuchsia miniskirt to a funeral or a tube top to temple. However, don't get hung up on the concept of "age-appropriate" either. Just because you've gone past fifty doesn't mean you have to wear brooches and *bubbe* shoes.

Speaking of shoes, most middle-aged women I know have traded in their spikes for something less likely to make them fall and break a hip. However, if you can hold yourself upright in high heels, knock yourself out (and I don't mean by diving head-first onto the dance floor).

Reprioritizing Friendship

⊰⊱

I was out to lunch with a couple of close girlfriends, one forty-seven and one fifty-seven. I asked them what was becoming more important to them at this stage of life and after a few minutes of brow wrinkling and table tapping, they came up with the same answer: friendship.

Both women had spent most of their lives working outside the home, both had been married for more than twenty years, both had raised children and/or stepchildren, both had done volunteer work and were active in their communities, both traveled extensively and both were active church goers. They were both financially secure and had at least one parent still alive. Yet, what they valued most as they entered midlife was communion with friends.

My mother told me this would happen. "Your friends are the ones who will be there for you at the finish line," she said.

At the risk of sounding like a Hallmark card or one of

those delightful chain e-mails that threaten you with death and dismemberment if you don't pass it on to eighteen associates within the next four minutes, friends do seem to ascend to a higher priority at midlife. Why?

You get to a point when work can only fulfill you so much. Your children grow to independence and leave, if you're lucky. Your spouse spends more time on the golf course than he does with you. The pool boy is getting long in the tooth. And, you may have fewer responsibilities and more time.

As you stagger down the unknown path of middle age, your youthful dreams have either come true or not. Now, you need to create new dreams. Friends help you keep things in perspective, opine on what they think you should do, accept your choices and catch you when you fall.

Old friends share your memories and reinforce that you have lived your life, for better or for worse. They knew you when. If they're still with you in the middle, they will probably be with you in the end—unless you have something that looks like it might be catching, in which case, they may keep their distance. They may move to another country entirely, but let's hope your real friends won't do that.

New friends bolster the notion that you still have much to offer, perhaps now more than ever. They sense your wisdom, your strength and, sometimes, your need.

Friends are on call to you twenty-four seven and enrich your life with their attention and their love. They're not in a hurry to rush to judgment because they've lived long enough to know that self-righteousness is counterproductive and their houses are made of glass, just like yours.

The best midlife friends:

- Tell you that you look great.

Let's face it. When you are approaching the change of life, your self-image changes, and not usually for the better. Most of the time, the change is so gradual, you barely notice that it's taking place. Maybe your weight has gone up and down your whole life. Maybe you've been coloring your hair since adolescence. Maybe the sun has already done a number on your complexion. You're accustomed to these changes.

The descent into midlife is subtler. You may begin to look like you haven't slept in a week. You may have bags under your eyes, lines forming around your mouth, and slackness in your neck and jaw line. You may not look the same in your jeans. This does not mean you are no longer beautiful. It means that your beauty has matured.

Youth isn't everything. If you think that it is, there's always plastic surgery. However, if youth is your only criterion for feeling attractive, your happiness will be skin-deep and short-lived. Take steps to keep healthy — physically, mentally, emotionally and spiritually — and try not to obsess over every little wrinkle. Self-acceptance at every stage of life will keep you beautiful and your good friends will tell you so. Believe them.

- Allow you to vent.

Life offers up all sorts of challenges. They're called "Little Murders." You've probably dealt with idiots, red tape and screw-ups your whole life. When you reach middle age, your tolerance for such matters is on a very short tether. When you're sleep-deprived, sweating, aching and bleeding three weeks out of every four, when your teenagers are flunking every subject including home room and your husband is sneaking off with his twenty-seven year old assistant, it's easy to get deranged when the roof blows off, the IRS comes a-calling and your cat has barfed in your handbag.

Sometimes, your upset can come from something as innocuous as someone accidentally cutting you off in a parking lot or a cashier innocently offering you a senior discount. What are they, out of their minds?

When moments such as these get you nettled beyond all human belief, your dear friends will listen to you and share your indignation—that is, unless they've had a lousy day themselves. Mutual venting doesn't do anyone much good. Hopefully, one of you will have the sense and sensitivity to yield the floor to the one who's in the greatest need at the moment. Your turn will come. There's no shortage of LMs out there.

• Offer you advice only when you ask for it.

Sometimes, all you want to do is rant. Hardly anyone likes unsolicited advice, but when you ask for it, that's another matter.

If you have a specific dilemma on your hands, a trusted friend may offer an opinion on how they would handle it or how they think you should handle it. Of course, their perspective may differ from yours, but their view may actually be clearer. Your thinking is probably muddled by emotion.

If you are asking for advice, be prepared to tell your confidante the whole story. If they only know half the facts, their response will only be relevant to half your problem.

- Can be trusted.

Obviously, it's important to know whom you can trust, at any stage of life. If you tell something to a friend in confidence, you want to know that your privacy is guaranteed. Some women think that their spouse is excluded from that pact. They are not. When you say, "Don't tell anyone," that includes your friend's husband, who probably doesn't give a damn about your secret anyway…unless it has something to do with him directly.

Your friend can also be trusted to tell you the truth (if you insist), not sleep with your teenaged son (unless you ask), provide comfort when needed (goes without saying) and not tempt you with coffee cake if you're on a diet (chocolate's a different story).

- Make you laugh.

Aging is no laughing matter, but if you can do it with a sense of humor, it will go a lot easier for you. Laughing is great therapy. The endorphin rush alone will make you feel years younger.

Having a friend who makes you laugh is a great gift. She (or he) doesn't have to be a stand-up comedian to crack you up over the sometimes-frightening vicissitudes of midlife, but it sure helps. Try having a good laugh with a puss full of Botox.

Now that would be funny.

Remember, laughing with a friend is good medicine. Laughing alone in a quiet room is psychotic and it scares the dog.

If you send this to eighteen of your closest friends within the next four minutes, your child will marry a doctor, you will find the world's greatest cosmetic surgeon and you will discover a cure for hot flashes that won't give you cancer. If you break the chain, you'll get crow's feet, vaginal atrophy and a visit from Babs.

Surviving Adversity

※❦※

*W*hat happens when you are in the throes of "the change" and adversity strikes? I'm not talking about trivial adversity like breaking a fingernail or accidentally dying your hair orange. I'm talking the big stuff like getting divorced after thirty years of marriage or developing cancer or skiing into a tree or—heaven forbid—all three.

How have you reacted to adversity in the past? Subtract from that a quart of estrogen and add a shot of maturity and you will have some idea of how you will respond to the green wienie when it's forced down your throat.

Consider the reliability of your support system. Many of those best buddies of yours will mysteriously disappear when you need them the most. People have a tendency to flee adversity, as if they're afraid it's contagious. What are you going to do when you're dealt a blow and you have no one to share it with except your cat? (Actually, pets can be a great source of unconditional love and compassion in a crisis, but they still can't sign for a Fed-Ex package, bring you chicken soup in bed or drive you to the oncologist.)

By the time we're fifty, most of us have had a taste of pain. If you are stricken down with an incapacitating illness and happen to be a control freak, your sanity is going to be sorely tested. People who survive trials best are those who accept there are some things they have no control over, take responsibility for what they do have control over, align themselves with people they can trust and have faith in the cyclical nature of fortune. Oh, and yes, those who have a particularly loving parakeet.

I've seen menopausal women get suicidal over an overcooked baked potato. On the other hand, I've seen menopausal women give birth in their mid-forties only to discover that their pregnancy activated the gene for breast cancer, which activates their husbands to leave—and these super women take all this in their stride (after an initial burst of hysteria—hey, they're entitled).

Attitude makes a huge difference in life. If you start out with a good attitude and carry it with you through middle age, you'll make out a lot better than your negative sisters.

It's easy to get depressed during midlife. Most of my female friends are on antidepressants because women are victims of mood-altering hormonal fluctuations from the time they reach puberty until the day they give up and wear red hats.

Middle age is particularly challenging because we are neither here nor there. We're basically beginning to cave in like overripe pumpkins.

Turns out, most popular antidepressants are just as dangerous as hormone replacement therapy, sometimes more so. Yet, doctors hand them out like candy. Believe me, you walk into a doctor's office and announce that you're fifty and the prescription pad comes out. I told my doctor that if he knew of a prescription antidepressant that wouldn't make me gain weight, lose my sex drive, keep me awake all night, give me a seizure or make me dizzy, homicidal or suicidal, I may give it a shot.

"Well, they all have side effects; you just have to experiment around a little," he said, pen poised in the air.

Experiment around with psychotropic drugs? I didn't like the sound of that. I took the scrip anyway—in case I got so desperately depressed, I no longer cared about side effects—an apathy that would likely be born from the side effect of inhaling carbon monoxide fumes in a closed garage.

Seriously, though, most of my friends have had good experience with psychotropic drugs until they've tried to wean themselves. That's when they take a big plunge into Crazyville. Sometimes, they end up on a ledge. Sometimes, they end up in a coma. I would have to be pretty deranged before I would risk either.

Of course, I haven't hesitated to pop herbal remedies like St. Johns's Wort for depression. It seems to work fine for mild to moderate melancholy but someday researchers may discover that long-term use of St. John's Wort makes your nose fall off. Nothing is risk free.

I've also tried SAMe, which is highly regarded by some physicians as a great mood enhancer, and good for arthritis and the liver, as well. Aside from a little stomach upset at high dosages, there are no known side effects. Unfortunately, in order to be truly effective for the typical midlife-size depression, you have to take a zillion pills a day. SAMe costs a small fortune and it is not covered by insurance. So, if you're a very wealthy depressed middle-aged woman with aches and pains and an old drinking habit, there's a great product on the market for you — no prescription required.

So, what do most of us do to comfort ourselves in the face of adversity? Do we just martyr ourselves and do nothing? Sometimes, it's the best thing to do, especially if our miseries are intermittent. If they're more chronic, something's got to give. Sometimes, we just have to bite the bullet and experiment with psychotropic drugs so we have a prayer of achieving a better balance and coping more effectively with whatever life has to offer up.

Just today, I was checking out some clothing in a department store when the cashier complained of her ever-worsening allergies.

"It's not just the allergies that have gotten worse," she said. "Everything just fell apart on me when I turned fifty."

"Tell me about it," I said, though I could see a line forming behind me.

"I can't take hormones because I have a history of cancer in my family," she began. "I was placed on Prozac. I got fat and couldn't lose the weight. Then, my husband divorced me. I was so depressed I couldn't get out of bed in the morning. The doctor took me off of Prozac and put me on Effexor. I feel a little better, but so what? I'm still alone and I can't get rid of the weight."

She had nice skin, at least.

I reassured her she was not alone. We exchanged numbers, and a mutually supportive relationship was formed. I could tell that the people waiting on line were thrilled for us.

Adversity seems to find us when we are at our weakest. Many middle-aged women are in a debilitated state, whether they're gambling with hormone replacement or not. They can maintain their beauty, their intelligence and their independence, but most women who approach fifty still require more reassurance than usual — much like thirteen-year-old girls.

Whether we get that reassurance from friends, spouses, doctors, lovers, counselors, pharmaceuticals, support groups or total strangers, it helps to know we're not alone and that a resurrection is possible on the other side of whatever chasm we've fallen into. We're at the beginning of a whole new path. Sometimes we need to help each other find it.

Is That All There Is?

*O*nce you have gone through menopause, you may wonder what else awaits you in life, aside from early-bird specials, senility and death — and not necessarily in that order. You begin to hear that old Peggy Lee song droning in your head: *Is That All There Is?* Hands down, it was the most depressing song ever written.

In a nutshell, the song is about a woman who is rescued from a house fire as a little girl, but doesn't find the fire all that thrilling; is taken to the circus at twelve, but can't get excited about it; has a bad breakup with a man as an adult and contemplates suicide but stops herself because she's in "no hurry for that final disappointment." Are you old enough to remember the refrain?

> *Is that all there is?*
> *Is that all there is?*
> *If that's all there is, my friends*

Then let's keep dancing
Let's break out the booze
And have a ball
If that's all there is.

Can you just die? I was very young when I first heard that song and already it made me feel like slashing my wrists. Peggy Lee looked like she had an injection of prehistoric Botox when she sang it, too. She crooned with the bland countenance of a Guernsey cow and the energy of a catatonic mental patient. I figured the song had to have been written by a woman in the middle of a monumental menopausal downer. Turns out, it was written by a couple of guys, Jerry Lieber and Mike Stoller.

Still, the answer is "No, that is not all there is," although it may seem like that sometimes. The point is that the woman survived the fire, was taken to the circus (not the dungeon) and experienced love—all good, life-affirming events, though fleeting. I'll bet that bottle of booze she broke out was half empty.

Life is a series of events, good and bad. It's hard to appreciate one without the other. By the time we reach midlife, we've had a pretty good dose of both. We begin to recognize that our time here is finite and we start to contemplate what happens when we leave— especially if we're not all that happy with the hand we've been dealt.

When I was young, I used to imagine all my loved ones lined up in caskets, gone from this life. It was an unbearable concept for me. It kept me up nights (that, and the memory of Peggy Lee's impassive *punam*). I would beg my father to reassure me that he would never die.

"I can't make you that promise because everything that lives will one day die," he said. Then, he added the words a fretful six-year-old insomniac didn't need to hear: "Even you."

Holy shit, I was going to die. Where would I go? How would I get there? Would I need a sweater? Would my turtles be there? Could I go barefoot? Who would do my homework? How would life go on without me? Even at six I was a solipsistic control freak.

All of these questions gave me something to chew on while my father left me alone so he could get some sleep. Of course, sleep was now out of the question for me. I began to have conversations with God.

These conversations were completely secular in nature. They were not in the form of prayer. I was never one to make deals with the Almighty, clasping my hands together on bended knee promising God I'd never tease my brother again if only He'd let me have the white ballet slippers with the pink ankle ribbons.

I had much bigger fish to fry when I spoke to the Guy in the Sky. I asked Him questions aloud and channeled His responses out of my own mouth. Our relationship was personal and intimate and I felt an intermingling of our spirits as I directed His energy through my own being. I was not subservient to this God. We were one. I was thus reassured that there was a lot more to me than braids and Cheerios and piano lessons, and that my life did not begin and end in this place and time.

Fast-forward forty years. By now, I have lost loved ones— grandparents, friends, pets—and I imagine I'm at least halfway to the finish line myself. I feel tightly connected to those who have predeceased me, and I speak to them much the same way I spoke to God as a child. I feel like they're to my left and right, above me and below me, living on a different plane. I do not see heaven and hell. I see coexistence. I'm comforted by their ethereal presence. They inform me in dreams and visions.

I also feel deeply conjoined with those who are still amongst the living. My relationships are not fleeting. Once begun, they never cease. I feel like I have gone through countless lives with the same group and sometimes I recognize someone upon meeting them for the first time. It's not an eerie sensation. It's an experience of familiarity, of joyful reunion, of perpetual love, of peace.

I am not a paranoid schizophrenic suffering from delusions. I actually did have a very meaningful conversation with my tuna fish sandwich this afternoon. (Only kidding—I had salmon.) I'm just a middle-aged woman who believes in eternal consciousness and the endurance of the soul.

As we age, we frequently reach out for something bigger than our work, our children, ourselves. Some of my friends have turned to religion. They find comfort in the rituals and reassurance that something more powerful than they is minding the store, so to speak. They enjoy the support of a like-minded community. Theirs' is a shared experience, and their collective spirit is moved by the sound of voices in unison.

Some of my friends throw a toothbrush and change of underwear into a daypack, check the dog into a kennel, tell their husbands they won't be home for dinner—and probably not for David Letterman either—shut off their cell phones and take off down the road, usually without a map. I have to admit, this takes a lot of guts but, if you survive, it's great for the spirit. For one day, you get to face down your fears—of being alone, of getting lost, of meeting strangers, of driving in the dark.

I took a spiritual journey on the first anniversary of the nine eleven terrorist attacks. I told my husband I was going to disappear for twenty-four hours to mourn the dead and celebrate life. He feared for my safety but didn't try to talk me out of it. He understands spiritual work and trusts my impulses.

I got into my car with a stiff neck and rapid pulse and started to drive. I was getting a late start. I put the car in charge. First it took me south. Then it took me east. I saw an exit sign for a town called Siloam. It looked like Shalom and I took that as a sign (actually, it was a sign). The road took me into the heart of backwoods Georgia, with long stretches of pine trees and pecan groves and tiny, whitewashed churches, one oddly bearing the Star of David.

I started to sing along with Diana Krall, love songs in Spanish. *Besame Mucho.* My neck started to relax and I felt perfectly secure. I didn't know where the hell I was, but the odometer told me I was more than a hundred miles from home. It could've just as easily been a thousand. I turned on my cell phone—no service. I wasn't merely alone; I was utterly alone.

It started getting dark, I kept driving on the two-lane road to nowhere. When the sky turned black and starry, I pulled over to gaze at the magnificent harvest moon with wisps of clouds drifting across its broad face. The air smelled of wood smoke. I nibbled on a chicken leg with Orion staring down at me from above. I spoke aloud to the spirits of the dead and they spoke back to me through the magnificence of this day. When their voices were replaced by the shrieks of coyotes, I knew it was time to get the flock out of there and end my journey. My car delivered me safely home.

If that's all there is, it's more than enough. But, what does it all mean?

I won't pretend to know the meaning of life here. We come into this world, either accidentally or intentionally, to fulfill someone's biological imperative.

When we're infants, we don't question our existence. We just are, and we are the center of the universe. When we're toddlers, the world still revolves around us, but we become more conscious of our effect on others. When we're young children, we can create heaven and hell for those around us, and we learn how to manipulate that power. When we're teenagers, we mostly live to create hell for others and ourselves. We spend most of our early adulthood realizing our potential, for better or for worse, and we may or may not fulfill our own biological imperative.

Then, along comes fifty. What's left for us to do aside from enjoy the thrill of the ride and the sight of a full moon in the dark country sky before fleeing the coyotes? Keep on dancing, my friends. The coyotes are getting closer.

Adjusting Your Attitude

֍

"*I* have no life."

If I had a nickel for every time I heard that phrase, I'd have at least a buck by now.

Having "no life" usually means having an abundance of life — too much work, too many children, too many commitments and too little help. The "no life" normally equates to "no time for you."

Most of us suffer from this condition because we are hard-driven, productive members of society who move forward like sharks. We feel guilty if we sit still for a minute. We mistake who we are with what we do.

Attitude accounts for a lot in life. If you are lucky enough to be born with a good nature, life will go a lot easier for you. Others may accuse you of being a Pollyanna, but that's their problem. If you came into the world angry, life can offer you the world on a platter, but you will never be satisfied. Most of us fall somewhere in the middle—with the occasional spectacular mood swing to remind us that we're chock full of female hormones.

It's important to not compare your life to anyone else's. We all have our own laughing place. Unfortunately, most of us think we want what others have.

When I was a nineteen-year-old college student, I worked as a cocktail waitress in the Borscht Belt. One night, as I was choking down a forkful of dry capon in the staff dining room, the manager came in and made an announcement.

He said, "If everyone in this room threw their package into the middle of the room, everyone would leap for their own package."

His words stuck to me through the decades (much like the capon stuck to my ribs) because they were both wise and true. I never coveted what was on someone else's plate.

My father put it another way. "Walk in your own shoes. If you try walking in somebody else's you may break your neck."

We make choices in life. Sometimes, they're made for us. Sometimes, luck is with us. Sometimes, it's not. If you disregard what you've got and pine for what you've not, you'll be crippled with regret and happiness will never find you.

When we're young, we fill our lives with work, with causes, with children, with empire building. We're too busy to have lunch with a friend, go to the spa, take a walk on the beach or read a book... we tell ourselves and others there'll be time enough for that when we're retired and the kids are grown.

We get exhausted and begin to resent the kids, the job, the husband, the in-laws and all the other people who are pulling pieces from us. We need to escape but we need the money, the prestige and the reinforcement more. What would we be without our various titles—president, doctor, consultant, mother, wife? What is left of us if all those identifications and responsibilities go away? Can less ever be more in this life? With the right attitude, yes, it can be ever so much more.

By the time we reach midlife, we are often forced to shift our goals and perspectives because we are changing in every way. It's extremely important to keep engaged with life, to have some purpose as we progress through time. Don't give up now. If you're lucky, you're only halfway down the road. It's time to regroup and reinvent, not retire and regret.

Your children will not be around forever. Your husband will not be around forever. Your career will not hold your interest forever. Your looks will change. Your energy level will diminish. Life will serve up all sorts of surprises, some good, some not. You will not always be able to look on the bright side. Your problems may seem petty in the grand scheme of things (losing a job or a fingernail is not in the same league as world hunger or an Ebola epidemic), but let's face it, we all feel our own pain and our feelings should not be trivialized — especially when we're a gallon low on estrogen.

If you're ready for a change (and I don't mean *the* change here — nobody's ready for that), you may want to consider the following:

- Don't commit the sin of omission or make excuses to keep from taking action. Life is a participant sport. You've got to show up.
- If you've made a commitment, don't be half-assed about it. Give it your heart and soul. If you get nothing in return within a reasonable time period, reconsider your options and get out if you can.
- Don't get hung up on yourself — it's not a good look for you. Others need your attention. Learn how to listen.

- Take responsibility for your actions and don't look to assign blame. Sometimes you just need to suck it up. If you're in the wrong, make amends and try to do better the next time.
- Don't have unreasonable expectations of others. Most people are very self-centered and can't see beyond their own noses. Realize that and make the appropriate adjustments in your thinking—but get rid of the chronically needy that only live to hear their own voices.
- Take the high road. It is possible to be a *mensch* without being a sucker.
- Love unconditionally, but know whom you're getting into bed with. There's no need to give until it hurts.
- Be more accepting of yourself. Your life may get smaller, but it may also get deeper, more concentrated and ultimately, richer and more fulfilling.
- Have a little faith. There may not be a pot of gold at the end of the rainbow, but the rainbow itself may be the reward.
- Try not to worry so much. As my chiropractor says, "If you can't eat it or screw it, piss on it." I don't know what that means, exactly, but my chiropractor believes thinking that way will help erase the frown lines from my forehead. (Yeah, that and a hypodermic needle full of Botox.)

Letting Go

⁂

*T*hink about all the time you waste fretting over things you can't control. Consider all the petty arguments, the feuds over real or imagined slights, the bickering over nonsense, the angry confrontations over trivia, the paranoia. Do you have any idea of what all this hostility does to your physical and mental health? Don't ask!

Apparently, human beings are very fragile. We're insecure. We're easily insulted. We look to find fault. We don't take responsibility. We shoot first and ask questions later. We're quick to feel persecuted. We have a drive to even the score. We tend to be righteous and judgmental. And, very few of us are capable of turning the other cheek, to say the least.

Almost invariably, we learn these behaviors from the people who raise us. We try not to pass on these crippling legacies, but we can't help ourselves. Our parents fucked us up one way. We'll fuck up our kids another way. Then, it'll be their turn. Nobody escapes. I don't mean to sound flip, but I see it occurring over and over again. We are pitifully lacking in love and compassion.

Couples argue over whose turn it is to answer the doorbell. Sisters stop speaking to each other because of ancient jealousies and misunderstandings. Friends part company because they stand on ceremony over who called who last. We avoid peaceful confrontation because we're afraid of expressing our feelings. Our rage festers until it explodes, leaving teeth, hair and eyeballs in its wake with no chance for reconciliation. Where does it all end?

We get sick. We end up ingesting a boatload of pharmaceuticals, which fix some problems and create others. We get bitter and bore people with endless diatribes about our troubles. We develop involutional melancholia and wallow in our regrets. Does that sound like the way you want to go?

Let's deal with control issues first. Most of us have a lot of balls in the air at once. We can't help it—it's the nature of life in the twenty-first century. Unless we have all eight arms, legs and eyes functioning at top efficiency at all times, those balls are going to start to spiral out of control. Multitasking becomes a little more challenging as we age. So, how do you keep it all together, especially when you get hit with the unexpected?

When life becomes unmanageable, make a list of everything you've got going on. Don't leave anything out. Draw a circle around everything on your list that you have any control over. You may as well cross out everything else. Situations that are beyond your control only serve to clutter your mind and deprive you of the energy you need to handle the events you do have control over.

The next step is to prioritize the items you have circled on your list. This isn't an easy task, but you're going to have to get good at it in order to regain control of your life. Through this exercise, you may choose to eliminate some items. Unless you have ADHD, paring down extraneous activity will make life more manageable and probably more productive, as well.

Once you have selected your "balls" wisely, assign a reasonable action plan and implementation timetable to each. Don't sign on for more than your plate can handle. Don't put anything off until *manana*. Take responsibility for everything on your list and execute your tasks to the best of your ability. What more can you do?

Letting go of hostility is also within your grasp.

Understand that you don't have control over anyone else's behavior. If you are accustomed to being a giver and you're confronted with an individual who is accustomed to being a taker, don't expect the taker to emulate your altruistic behavior. If you have that expectation, you are going to be disappointed, and worse. You're going to come to resent the hell out of that taker, and they're just being themselves.

You are a giver either by nature, by goodness, by love, by duty or by ulterior motive. The latter is a closet taker, by the way... someone who gives with the intention of taking back a lot more, sooner or later.

Very few of us are pure givers, even if we have the best of intentions. After a while, we feel like we're firing squash balls into space. If we are dealing with the relentlessly selfish, the unpardonably ungrateful, the nauseatingly spoiled, the inexcusably rude or those who feel eternally entitled, our graciousness will begin to wear thin. And, it should. Get a grip on your self-respect and cut the selfish bastards loose. I don't care who they are. You're not a doormat, for Christ's sake.

Stop sweating the small stuff. You've heard that expression before. There should be no debate over whose turn it is to answer the door. When the doorbell rings, get off your ass and answer it. If someone has upset you repeatedly, don't keep them guessing about why you've clammed up. Nobody is served by a breakdown in communication. Tell them how you feel. If they respond with defensiveness, angry rebuttal or ridicule, what's your relationship worth? Not much. Let them go.

You are not immune to being a jerk, by the way. Sometimes, you're in the wrong and you need to acknowledge it and atone for it. In this case, you are letting go of your own self-righteousness and pride and accepting that you're human enough to make a mistake. Fess up, make amends and let it go. If the wronged party can't forgive you—if they are, in fact, full of small-mindedness or Biblical wrath, let them go. You don't need to be around someone with an axe to grind. Life's too short.

Here's a practical list of other things to let go of:

- Trying to change someone's religion or politics. These are highly personal areas and it's not your business to force your agenda down someone else's throat. Let it go.
- Trying to break someone else's addictions. Most addicts care more about the monkeys on their backs than they care about you. They need to get to a point of personal crisis before they quit whatever it is they're addicted to. At that time, they make a decision about whether they want to live or die, and you have little to do with that decision. Let it go.
- Trying to make somebody love you. If someone is inclined to love you, you can behave horrendously and they will probably still love you. If someone is disinclined to love you,

you can bend over backwards and still not win their love. Let it go.

- Reasoning with idiots. If you've ever tried reasoning with an idiot you will find it bears a striking resemblance to banging your head against the wall. Let it go.

- Lying about your age. When I was little, my grandmother convinced me she was a year younger than my mother. My mother, in turn, always told people she was a year younger than she actually was—until it was time to collect Social Security, at which time, the fib became counterproductive. Good thing, too—I was on the verge of being older than both of them. Who are we kidding when we lie about our age? Nobody. Let it go.

- Feelings of immortality. No matter how many supplements we take, no matter how many times we have our faces and butts lifted, no matter how many glasses of water we drink, no matter how many times we redecorate the living room, no matter how many times we pump iron, no matter how much money we've got, we're all going to die someday. Accept it. And, let it go.

Accepting the Change

When I was in college, I had a flawlessly beautiful roommate named Violette. She had the magnificent facial structure of a Greek goddess, creamy skin, high cheekbones, almond-shaped blue eyes, thick chestnut-colored hair, Patrician nose and perfect white teeth. Ironically, she looked just like her father. The only thing she got from her mother was a nice ass. Of course, there's something to be said for that, too.

Violette was a wonderful artist. One day, she presented me with a picture she had drawn of herself. "This is me at fifty", she said.

The drawing focused on her face only. It was Violette, all right, but it looked like all her features were in the process of melting. Her almond eyes now looked more like walnuts, heavily lidded above and puffy beneath. There were creases in her forehead, deep furrows along both sides of her mouth, her regal nose had headed south and her chin seemed to blend into her neck. She wasn't smiling, and with good reason. I sure hoped she looked better from behind.

I looked at her in dismay. "What kind of a life have you been leading?" I asked.

Violette's parents were both under forty, so she wasn't taking any cues from them. Maybe she felt like she would finally pay the price for not eating her vegetables or smoking her dietetic cigarettes (those "lite" jobbies that taste like Vicks VapoRub).

Violette didn't share my horror. She maintained an artistic detachment from her subject matter. Her exaggeratedly aged visage may have just as easily been a still life of rotting fruit. But, Violette was all right with that. She accepted the inevitability of physical decline and exaggerated it to the nth degree.

How are fifty-year-old women typically portrayed? I'm talking about women who have not been surgically altered and puffed up like Christmas geese.

The words, "handsome" and "well-preserved" come to mind, especially if the woman was formerly beautiful. More often than not, middle-aged women are described as "distinguished," "sturdy," "hardy," "tough" or, God forbid, "matronly."

When was the last time you heard a woman of fifty plus described as "hot" —aside from when she was having a flash? Even Mrs. Robinson, the middle-aged seductress in *The Graduate*, was eventually reviled by her young lover as a "broken down alcoholic," and then abandoned as he runs off with her nubile daughter.

Feisty fifty-year-olds do abound in the media but are made to look ridiculous, pathetic or downright predatory, like the appalling Martha in *Who's Afraid of Virginia Woolf?*.

I recently read Michael Cunningham's *The Hours*, a book about three different generations of women, all confronting death one way or the other. He wrote several passages regarding middle-aged women.

One portrays Clarissa, a character in her early fifties, played by Meryl Streep in the movie version.

"She looks older, Louis thinks in astonishment. It's finally happening. What a remarkable thing, these genetic trip wires, the way a body can sail along essentially unaltered, decade after decade, and then in a few years capitulate to age."

Another tells how a younger female, played by Toni Collette, will descend—or, rather, crash—into midlife.

"She seems, briefly, like a simple, ordinary woman seated at a kitchen table. Her magic evaporates; it is possible to see how she'll look at fifty—she'll be fat, mannish, leathery, wry and ironic about her marriage, one of those women of whom people say, 'She used to be quite pretty, you know.' The world is already, subtly, beginning to leave her behind."

Another passage describes how Clarissa envisions her teenaged daughter, played by Claire Danes, at fifty.

"She will be what people refer to as an ample woman, large of body and spirit, inscrutably capable, decisive, undramatic, an early riser."

We are programmed from puberty to accept natural aging as patently unattractive, and this debilitating mindset is constantly being reinforced in the media. This is so terribly wrong. Regardless of whether our faces are smooth or wrinkled, regardless of whether our breasts turn up or down, we all need to be loved, we all need reassurance that we are valued, and we all want to be desired and touched.

My husband told me, "One of the reasons I married you was because I knew you'd be beautiful forever—not because of your appearance but because of your presence."

Appearance relates to the façade, the skin. We do whatever we can to preserve that skin, but, no matter how many emollients we apply, no matter how many times we nip and tuck, the skin eventually betrays us.

Presence is a far more enduring trait. It means charisma, allure, appeal and magnetism. Presence suggests power that transcends age and worldly appearance, and that's sexy. And, I sure prefer sexy to dignified or handsome.

When you imagine yourself at fifty, regardless of whatever discomfort you may experience as you go through this awesome change, remember the power of your presence. It's made of courage, playfulness, intelligence, a sense of humor and the ability to love completely.

Walk with purpose, smile often and carry yourself like you're proud. You can look beautiful at any age. And, if you put some effort into keeping healthy and fit, your exterior will look better, too. In fact, you may end up looking better at fifty than at any other time in your life.

How do you see yourself? Two generations ago, fifty looked like Granny Clampett. Last generation, it looked like Dyan Cannon playing the beautiful "wattled" Judge Whipper on *Ally McBeal*. Nowadays, it could look like the confident, elegant Diane character on *The Good Wife*, played by Christine Baranski, or it could look like Cher, complete with feathers, rhinestones and collagen injections. Will future generations strive to tighten themselves until there's not an inch of skin left to stretch?

Preconceived notions of how we're supposed to look and behave at fifty heavily influence the way we see ourselves. This happens at every stage of life.

When we're teenagers, we look and behave in ways to attract

a mate. Once we have found a mate and achieved maternity, we become sainted mothers with varicose veins and hemorrhoids, and many of our partners are drawn to less sacred sex objects (i.e., women whose breasts have not yet been converted to milk bottles).

Then, midlife comes along and the only time we're seen jumping for joy is when we've discovered a new drug for hot flashes that may or may not kill us. We're not viewed as sex objects anymore, which is too bad because we're at a time when we could really use some affirmation of our sexuality and femininity.

There's nothing wrong with behaving grandmotherly. There's nothing wrong with being a senior board member. There's nothing wrong with being called "ma'am" (in the South, that happens by the time you reach twenty-five). There's nothing wrong with wearing sensible shoes. There's nothing wrong with fanning yourself in public. Just don't ever forget that you're a woman, and will be until your dying day (or until the day you decide it's not worth it and start taking testosterone shots).

Preparing for the Back Fifty

✥

*S*omeday, when you least expect it, the *schvitzing* will stop. You will have completed your trip over the rainbow and returned home to your black and white world again, a little older, a little wiser, a little happier for finally vanquishing the Wicked Witch of the Wretched (aka menopause). You will wake up on fabulously dry sheets after a full night of blissfully undisturbed sleep, look into the mirror with a big smile on your face and exclaim, "Holy shit, I'm ancient!"

Hey, what did you expect? You've just gone through several years of torment and now have the estrogen count of a Hostess Twinkie—except if you've been on HRT all these years, in which case you look and feel a lot better than most of us—unless you're dead.

Now it's time to get on with the rest of your life while dodging the many diseases and maladies that bedevil older women (yes, that would be you), not including tripping over your own wattle. Does that sound like a daunting task? It is.

Aging is not for sissies, but you have to assume it's better than the alternative. Speaking of which, maybe we should all have a shot of embalming fluid on the rocks – it lasts longer than Botox.

Enough tomfoolery. I didn't lead you all the way to this final chapter to leave you with no hope. Here are some words of encouragement: The back fifty can be better than the front fifty. (If you believe that, I've got a nice piece of swampland in Georgia for you! Okay, I promise, no more kidding.)

Think about all you couldn't accomplish in the first half of your life. You put off doing what you wanted to do because you had too little time or too many kids or too little money or too much work. You devoted your energies to building careers or families, or both. Now, it's time for you.

Wisdom is supposed to be the big prize of aging. If we are savvy enough to pay attention to all that life has taught us to date, we have a crack at real happiness going forward. We should also observe and listen closely to our elders. Their wisdom has had a chance to ferment longer than ours and should be taken seriously. Everybody's experience is different, but each experience counts and can give us valuable insights into what works and what doesn't.

Here are a few things I've learned over the years:

- The happiest people I know are excited about their work. If you love your work and have the stamina to continue with it, do not retire.
- Keep mentally alert. If you don't want to work until your dying day, take on a hobby that keeps your mind busy – like cards or crossword puzzles or reading.

- Keep busy. Active people don't have the time to worry about how old they're getting. Find something you love to do and do it.
- Do volunteer work. Giving freely to others is very life affirming and it makes you realize that there are worse things in life than frown lines.
- Surround yourself with positive, upbeat people who don't try to rob you of your energy at every opportunity.
- Take up meditation. It doesn't matter what kind. You don't even have to sit in a meditation posture. Just close your eyes and take a break from the world's noise for a few minutes each day.
- Eat healthfully, but don't begrudge yourself the occasional excess. Telling yourself you're eating poison every time you put a goody in your mouth will not only ruin your experience — it will ruin everybody else's experience as well.
- Try not to harp on your physical maladies. Yes, they will become a bigger and bigger part of your life, but dwelling on them will not make them go away. Take steps to relieve your pain.
- I'm not suggesting you run a marathon, but do try to keep as physically active as possible. It will make you feel and look better. Twiddling your thumbs doesn't count as exercise.
- Keep culturally active. Even if you're on oxygen, you can still enjoy live theater (unless you've hated it in the past, in which case something like *Les Miserables* may kill you).
- Always strive to look your best. Aging is no reason to give up on attractiveness. Avoid hats and clothing that scream, "Dowager Club," unless they truly give you pleasure.
- Keep socially active. Unless you prefer the life of a hermit,

interacting with others can be stimulating and enjoyable (unless they're always telling you what not to eat or only want to hear the sound of their own voice).

- Don't impose an age restriction on sex. Have it as long and as often as you can. If you die, you die.
- Don't stop exploring the world, even if you do get strip-searched at airports.
- Understand that we are all just aging children. Never lose your sense of wonder.
- If you can't stand to look in the mirror, either lose the mirror or change your appearance.
- Take inventory of your life's accomplishments and figure out what else you would like to do. Having a sense of purpose will keep you going.

As I finished writing this book, I completed my fiftieth year and, since I practice what I preach, I took inventory of the highlights of the past year.

I celebrated my birthday in Hawaii. I wore a string bikini on the beach. At the very least, it kept the sharks away. On the trip, my husband and I flew in and out of at least eight airports. I got frisked at every single checkpoint, but it was worth it. The TSA agents apparently double as masseuses.

I've been operating a successful business since nineteen eighty-seven. This year, I gave myself a break so I could clear my head and think about what else I would like to do. My mind is open. Who knows what will drop into it. Hopefully, nobody will mistake it for a urinal.

Somebody actually did manage to sell me a piece of swampland in Georgia. At the same time, somebody else sold me a forty thousand dollar well on my property in Santa Fe. I guess it's all about water, the source of all life. In one case, it'll probably come through the second-story windows. In the other, it'll have to be dredged up from China. Next year, I may invest in a polar ice cap in Greenland. It's good to have a plan.

I joined a health club and began to feel very strong and fit until my back went out. That's when I discovered that a standard sports bra could double as a traction device.

The most enjoyable thing I did all year was to write this book. It helped me put my whole life in perspective and got me hooked on green tea, which I understand retards cellular degeneration. Yeah, tell that to my jaw line.

If sixty is the new thirty, it follows that fifty is the new twenty. That makes me twenty-one plus (yes, I'm officially past fifty) — old enough to drink, vote, marry and make stupid mistakes in most of the civilized world (wherever that is, these days). What am I going to do with this great, big life that lies ahead of me?

A psychic told me I would give birth to a daughter at fifty-three. I'm a bit of a seer myself and I predict that I will give birth when hell turns into an orange Popsicle. No, my future will have nothing to do with changing diapers, unless they're my own.

My future will have little to do with worldly preoccupations. I will continue to pay the bills and go for annual Pap tests and scarf down massive quantities of vitamins and check my e-mails; but, when I emerge from my chrysalis, I will have a far greater appreciation for what lies beyond the tiny space which is my physical life.

For those of you who are just turning fifty, I hope this book has been of some use to you. I wish you the best year of your life, and who knows what wonders await in the future. Here's a little song to get you started. Sing it to the tune of *Makin' Whoopee*.

It's very clear
That this girl here
Is turning fifty
This very year
She's got the gray hair
But what does she care
She's turning fifty
She can't read close
She can't run far
Her teeth are sleeping
In a glass jar
She can't remember
If it's December
Because she's fifty
What's there to do?
What can you say?
When all your forties
Have gone away?
My words are thrifty
I think it's nifty
She's turning fifty

CPSIA information can be obtained at www.ICGtesting.com
Printed in the USA
LVOW041746261111

256570LV00003B/10/P